Forensic Medicine and Toxicology

Log Book-cum-Practical Manual

Name of the Student ____

College/Institute ____

Class Roll No. _____________________ Session/Year_____________

University Roll No. ____

Forensic Medicine and Toxicology

Log Book-cum-Practical Manual

As per the Revised Competency Based Medical Education Curriculum of NMC

SECOND EDITION

Gautam Biswas MD (UCMS)

Professor and Head
Department of Forensic Medicine and Toxicology
Dayanand Medical College and Hospital
Ludhiana, Punjab, India

Forewords

Pramod Tiwari

Deepak Sharma

Sangeet Dhillon

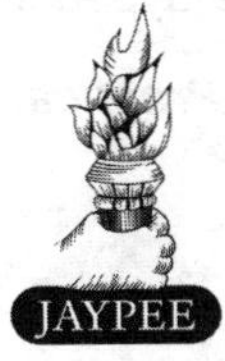

JAYPEE BROTHERS MEDICAL PUBLISHERS

The Health Sciences Publisher

New Delhi | London

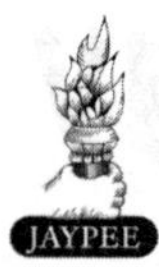 **Jaypee Brothers Medical Publishers (P) Ltd**

Headquarters

EMCA House
23/23-B, Ansari Road, Daryaganj
New Delhi 110 002, India
Landline: +91-11-23272143, +91-11-23272703
+91-11-23282021, +91-11-23245672
E-mail: jaypee@jaypeebrothers.com

Corporate Office

Jaypee Brothers Medical Publishers (P) Ltd.
4838/24, Ansari Road, Daryaganj
New Delhi 110 002, India
Phone: +91-11-43574357
Fax: +91-11-43574314
E-mail: jaypee@jaypeebrothers.com

Overseas Office

JP Medical Ltd.
83, Victoria Street, London
SW1H 0HW (UK)
Phone: +44-20 3170 8910
E-mail: info@jpmedpub.com

EU GPSR Authorised Representative

Logos Europe, 9 rue Nicolas Poussin
17000, La Rochelle, France
Phone: +33 (0) 6 67 93 73 78
E-mail: Contact@logoseurope.eu

Website: www.jaypeebrothers.com
Website: www.jaypeedigital.com

Inquiries for bulk sales may be solicited at: jaypee@jaypeebrothers.com

Forensic Medicine and Toxicology: Log Book-cum-Practical Manual

First Edition: 2021
Second Edition: 2024
Revised Reprint: **2025**

ISBN: 978-93-5696-924-7

Printed in India by Rajkamal Electric Press, Kundli, Haryana-131 028.

Dedicated
to
My teachers
&
All my students—Past, Present and Future

'Tell me and I'll forget. Show me and I'll remember. Involve me and I'll understand'

—Confucius

Foreword

The previous edition of this practical manual by Dr Gautam Biswas was undoubtedly a great work created with perfection, but the updated *"Forensic Medicine and Toxicology: Log Book-cum-Practical Manual"* in its 2nd edition which has been restructured as per the demands of the National Medical Commission's Competency Based Medical Education (CBME) is an "absolute gem". Although intended for undergraduates, it shall serve well to postgraduates as a ready reference and will be useful for upcoming National Exit Test (NEXT) which is expected to put emphasis on practical skills. It shall also be usable in various medical universities/colleges across India as the book is well structured into diverse sections which give due weightage to skill-based learning and self-directed learning which appeared in the amended Regulations on Graduate Medical Education (GMER) 2019.

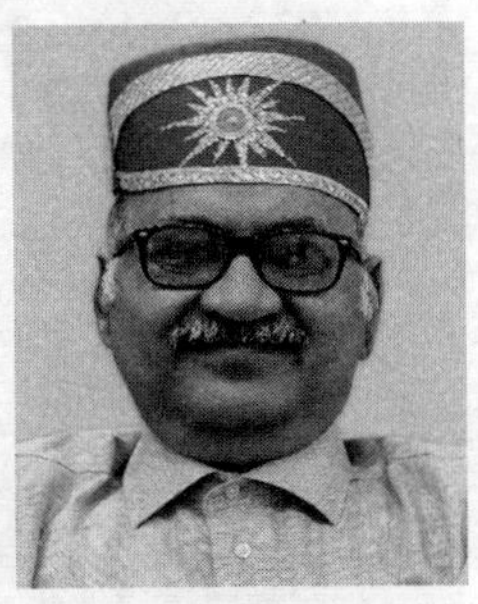

There is a separate section on Attitudes, Ethics, and Communication (AETCOM) module which will lessen the prevailing confusion and help the medical teachers in the better implementation of the new medical curriculum. This will also serve the purpose of a log book to document the progress of the medical student in relation to practical skills and special learning modules. The book has a user-friendly way of presentation which makes it easier to follow the practical demonstration and hence acquire the intended psychomotor and intellectual skills.

The model proformas and sample medicolegal/postmortem reports shall be further useful for Medical Officers and shall also serve as a guide for the students. Exercises in Clinical Forensic Medicine and colored photographs of medicolegal aspects of injuries, toxicological specimens, and histopathological slides will be useful for medical students.

The last section on simulation-based teaching and vertical integration in Forensic Medicine will make the subjected interesting and be relatable to the undergraduates who will appreciate the legal implications of medical findings, whether be it in a civil or a criminal context.

Wishing all the Success.

Pramod Tiwari
Senior Professor and Head of Forensic Medicine
Principal and Controller
Government Medical College
Chittorgarh, Rajasthan, India

Foreword

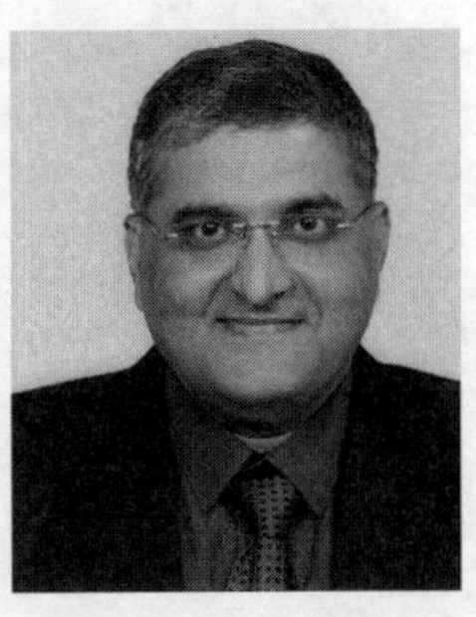

It gives me immense pleasure and pride to pen down the foreword for the book *"Forensic Medicine and Toxicology: Log Book-cum- Practical Manual, 2nd edition"*. Clinical Forensic Medicine holds its own significance in every medico's life. As I turn every page of this book, I observed how this book is customized as per the Competency Based Medical Education (CBME) guidelines which makes it easy and interesting for the students to learn. In this Logbook cum Practical Manual, the author has tried to cover every nook and corner of the practical aspect of Forensic Medicine under four different Sections. With the innovative exercise "Project" every student will be trained strong in the medicolegal aspects and together we can cater to the medicolegal needs of society in a better way. This book has incorporated various Skill-based training modules, self-directed learning (SDL), AETCOM, and stimulation-based training (Skill Lab) as recommended by the National Medical Commission. As a Professor of Forensic Medicine, I believe that this book will marvel as an inseparable companion during the MBBS and even for their future legal practices. With the explosion of knowledge and ongoing curricular changes, this manual has been revised and more student friendly. The objectives are well defined, and the language is simplified so that it can be comprehended by one and all. With the evolving concept of "Adult Learning Principles", i.e., Adults learn from what they "DO" and the global movement toward the "competency-based curriculum", this manual will help the students to become competent doctors.

Dr Gautam Biswas, is a well-renowned teacher and an eminent writer. Knowing him personally for the last 10 years, I really appreciate his enthusiasm and interest in educating the upcoming generations. I wish him and his team to continue their elite work and bring light in the life of students.

Deepak Sharma
Member, National Medical Commission
Professor, Department of Forensic Medicine
Government Medical College, Kota, Rajasthan, India

Foreword

It is honor and privilege for me to introduce the book *Forensic Medicine and Toxicology: Log Book-cum-Practical Manual*, 2nd edition by Dr Gautam Biswas. This practical manual has been changed and modified according to the new competency-based medical education guidelines for Indian Medical Graduates of National Medical Commission (NMC), thus covering the prescribed practicals.

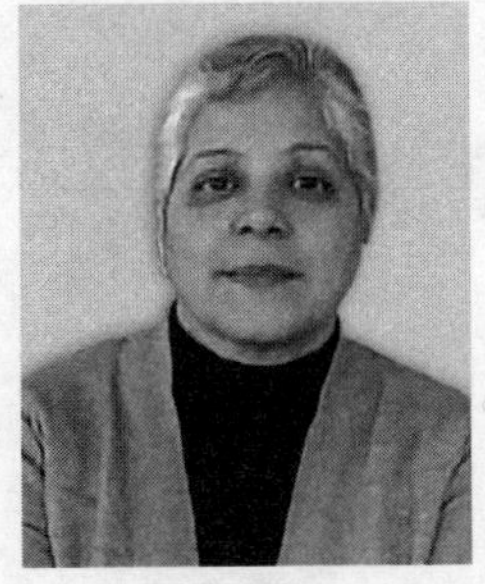

Further, not only practicals are covered, it also has other sections such as SDL, AETCOM, and simulation-based teaching making the manual a complete practical book. This will not only help the students to complete the syllabus but also help in developing an interest in the subject and be more confident in day-to-day administration work when the students get to work on the post of medical officer.

The model proformas and sample medicolegal/postmortem reports shall be further useful for Medical Officers and shall also serve as a guide for the students. Exercises in Clinical Forensic Medicine and colored photographs of medicolegal aspects of injuries, toxicological specimens, and histopathological slides will be useful for medical students.

The last section on simulation-based teaching and vertical integration in Forensic Medicine will make the subjected interesting and be relatable to the undergraduates who will appreciate the legal implications of medical findings, whether be it in a civil or a criminal context.

Wishing all the Success.

Sangeet Dhillon
Professor and HOD
Department of Forensic Medicine
Dr YSP Government Medical College
Nahan, Himachal Pradesh, India

Preface to the Second Edition

It gives me immense pleasure to introduce the all new and revised *Forensic Medicine and Toxicology: Log Book-cum-Practical Manual (2nd edition)* to the undergraduate students. The new Competency Based Graduate Medical Education (CBME) regulations have been implemented by the medical colleges all over India. During the period of 2 years spanning across II MBBS and Final Part I MBBS, the CBME suggested a number of skills that must be developed/performed independently by the students and participate actively in Self-Directed Learning (SDL) and Attitude, Ethics and Communication (AETCOM). The skills need to be assessed in the practical laboratory, skills laboratory, and skills station that uses mannequins/paper case/simulated patients/real patients as the context demands. The same is to be documented and certified in his/her log book. The purpose of the manual is to provide guidelines to the students as well as to the teachers to achieve defined outcomes in this subject through learning and assessment.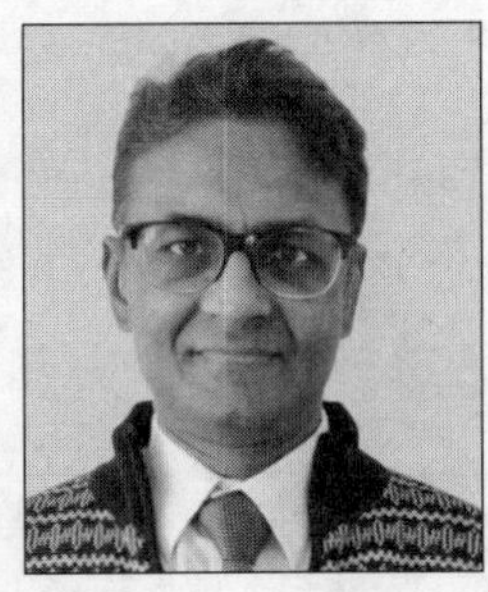

The book comprises four sections—first section deals with skills, second is about SDL, third is about AETCOM, and fourth requires documentation on Simulation Based Teaching (Skill Lab), Vertical Integration, and Seminars.

The material in "Skills" includes hypothetical case-based studies, which will give the students an overview and understand the various scenarios that they may encounter practically. Each worksheet has been carefully drafted to help the students get a thorough insight into the topic. There are 15 proformas for postmortem examination, color photographs for the injuries, preservation of trace evidence, X-rays for age estimation, death certification, toxicological specimens, and histopathogical slides. Sample medicolegal report, postmortem report, and death certificate have been included for better understanding of these practicals. However, the students should have a sound knowledge regarding the cases they are dealing with, and to finalize the report, they should come well prepared for the practicals and actively participate in them. There is a separate unit on "writing a case report (Project)" which will give an exposure to the budding minds in clinical forensic medicine.

The teachers/faculty members on their part will have to guide the students in filling up the proformas, which are self-explanatory in most aspects. The teachers may use the short case history given along with the proformas or may give a separate case scenario. If more than one exercise of the same topic needs to be done, then a photocopy of the same may be obtained. The reflections on SDL, AETCOM, Simulation Based Teaching (Skill Lab), Vertical Integration, and Seminars can be filled up as per the teaching program and curriculum of that college.

It is hoped that this book fills the vacuum for a standardized practical notebook, as well as log book in the subject of Forensic Medicine and Toxicology, which will bring uniformity throughout the country as to the implementation of National Medical Commission (NMC) guidelines. It is also hoped that this book will get a favorable response from the faculty like my previous book "Manual of Practical Forensic Medicine and Toxicology" and that they will not hesitate in recommending the same to their students.

Gautam Biswas

Preface to the First Edition

It gives me immense pleasure to present the *Manual of Practical Forensic Medicine and Toxicology* to the undergraduate students. The new Competency Based Graduate Medical Education (CBME) Regulations have been implemented by the medical colleges all over India. The subject of Forensic Medicine and Toxicology is now spanned over two professionals—2nd MBBS and Final MBBS Part (1) with examination to be held after completion of Final MBBS Part (1). During this period of 2 years, the CBME suggested a number of skills that must be developed/performed independently by the student and the same to be certificated in his/her log book. The skill need to be assessed in the practical laboratory, skills laboratory, skills station that uses mannequins/paper case/simulated patients/real patients as the context demands. The purpose of the manual is to provide guidelines to the students, as well as to the teachers to achieve defined outcomes in this subject through learning and assessment. All the competencies mentioned in the index for the training of 2nd MBBS and Final MBBS (Part 1) students are to be documented in the manual.

In addition to competencies suggested by the MCI, this edition covers almost all the medico-legal cases/issues which the student may encounter during his/her professional career. The material includes hypothetical case-based studies, which will give the students a practical overview and understand various scenarios that they may encounter, and photographs including X-rays. Each worksheet has been carefully drafted to help the students get a thorough insight of the topic. In this edition, 15 proformas for postmortem examination, color plates for the injuries, toxicological specimens and histopathogical slides have been included as per the recent CBME guidelines of the MCI. There is a separate unit on 'writing a case report (Project)' which will give an exposure to the budding minds in clinical forensic medicine. However, the students should have a sound knowledge regarding the cases they are dealing with, and to finalize the report, they should come well prepared for the practicals and actively participate in them.

The teachers/faculty members on their part will have to guide the students in filling up the proformas, which are self-explanatory in most aspects. The teachers may use the short case history given along with the proformas or may give a separate case scenario. If more than one exercise of the same topic needs to be done, then a photocopy of the same may be obtained.

It is hoped that this practical manual fills the vacuum for a standardized notebook, which is a need of the hour for the undergraduates. It is also hoped that this book will get a favorable response from the faculty like my previous book "Practical and Postmortem Record Book of Forensic Medicine and Toxicology" and that they will not hesitate in recommending the same to their students.

Gautam Biswas

Acknowledgments

I would like to place on record my deepest gratitude and respect to all my teachers who played a significant role in mentoring me.

Dr Aminder Singh (Associate Professor, Department of Pathology) and Dr Devinder Pal Singh (Assistant Professor, Department of Radiology), DMCH, Ludhiana, Punjab, India, deserve special mention and thanks for providing logistic support. I am grateful to Dr Viswakanth B, Dr Murugesa Bharathi, Dr Rajendra Singh Kulhari, Dr Sandip Mukhopadhyay, Dr Mohit Gupta, Dr Anil Kohli, Dr Lishu Chuare, Dr Vivek Kumar, Dr Parmod Goyal, Dr Amarjyoti Patowary, Dr Jitender Kumar Jakhar, and Dr Abhishek Das for the images in the section on "Injuries".

My deepest respect and gratitude go out to Shri Bipin Gupta, Secretary, Managing Society, DMCH; Dr Sandeep Puri, Principal; Dr GS Wander, Vice-Principal; and Dr Sandeep Kaushal, Dean, DMCH, for their continuous support, motivation, and encouragement. I would also like to express my sincerest thanks to Dr Virendar Pal Singh, my friend and colleague, for supporting and encouraging me during this venture. I wish to express my thanks to Dr Varun Modgil, Senior Resident, PGI Chandigarh for helping me whenever required.

I would like to express my heartfelt thanks to the following faculty members for providing valuable suggestions, encouragement, and support—Dr SK Verma and Dr Anil Kohli (University College of Medical Sciences and Guru Teg Bahadur Hospital, Delhi), Dr Suresk K Dhattarwal and Dr Jitender Kumar Jakhar (Post Graduate Institute of Medical Sciences, Rohtak), Dr Dasari Harish (Government Medical College and Hospital, Chandigarh), Dr Mukul Chopra (Punjab Institute of Medical Sciences, Jalandhar), Dr Mukta Rani (Lady Hardinge Medical College, New Delhi), Dr Sunil Naagar (MAMC, Delhi), Dr Ashok Moondra (GMC, Kota), Dr Baljit Singh Khurana (Sri Guru Ram Das Medical College, Amritsar), Dr RK Mathur (JLN Medical College, Ajmer, Rajasthan), Dr Bhupesh Khajuria (GMC, Kathua, Jammu and Kashmir), Dr Aditya Sharma (IGMC, Shimla, HP), Dr Vijay Arora and Dr Susheel Sharma (GMC, Tanda, HP), Dr Rajiv Joshi (Government Medical College, Faridkot), Dr Aakashdeep Aggarwal (Government Medical College, Patiala), Dr Deepak Sharma (MMU, Solan, Himachal Pradesh), Dr Pooja Rastogi (School of Medical Sciences and Research, Greater Noida, UP), Dr Sandhya Arora (Government Medical College and Hospital, Jammu), Dr Swapnil S Agarwal (Pramukhswami Medical College, Anand), Dr JP Singh (Noida International Institute of Medical Science), Dr Sandesh Chaudhari (CCMMC, Chhattisgarh), and Dr Tarun Dagar (Dr Radhakrishnan Government Medical College, Hamirpur).

I want to express my deepest gratitude to M/s Jaypee Brothers Medical Publishers (P) Ltd, New Delhi, India, for their acceptance in publishing the work and their professionalism during the entire process. I am especially grateful to Shri Jitendar P Vij (Group Chairman), Mr Ankit Vij (Managing Director), Mr MS Mani (Group President), Dr Madhu Choudhary (Director–Educational Publishing), Ms Pooja Bhandari [Director–Production (Books and Journals)], Ms Sunita Katla (Executive Assistant to Group Chairman and Publishing Manager), Mr Ajay Kumar Sharma [Deputy General Manager (Books and Journals)], Ms Samina Khan (Executive Assistant to Director–Educational Publishing), Mr Rajesh Sharma (Production Coordinator), Ms Seema Dogra (Cover Visualizer), Ms Neelam Kakriya (Proof Reader), Mr Dinesh Bhardwaj (Typesetter), Mr Sumit Kumar (Graphic Designer), for shaping up of the manual and making all the changes, without any complaints.

This work would not have been possible without the blessing of the Almighty and unconditional love and support of my family. I would like to express my love and gratitude to my dearest son Gaurav and wife Anupama, for their patience, constant support, and encouragement. My apologies to all my colleagues, friends, and students whose names I have omitted inadvertently.

Certificate

This is to certify that the candidate Mr/Ms____,
Reg. No. ___________, admitted in the year ___________ in _______________________
Medical College, _________________, has satisfactorily completed/has not completed all
assignments/requirements mentioned in this manual for 2nd MBBS and Final MBBS
(Part I) course in the subject of Forensic Medicine and Toxicology during the period from
_______________ to__________.

She/He is/is not eligible to appear for the summative (University) assessment as on the
date given below.

____

Signature of Faculty

Name and Designation

Countersigned by Head of the Department

Principal/Dean of the College

Place: _______________________

Date: _______________________

Log Book in Forensic Medicine and Toxicology

Sub Item: Certificates/Medico-legal reports/Museum session/Postmortem examination/ Early clinical exposure/ Vertical integration/Seminar/Self-directed Learning

1	2	3	4	5	6	7	8
Competency addressed	Name of activity	Date completed (dd-mm-yyyy)	Attempt at activity First or only (F) Repeat (R) Remedial (Re)	Rating Below (B) expectations Meets (M) expectations Exceeds (E) expectations	Decision of faculty Completed (C) Repeat (R) Remedial (Re)	Initial of faculty and date	Feedback received (Initial of learner)

(This table can be replicated in as many pages in log book, as needed)

Explanation of each Column in the Log Book Table

1. The number of the competency addressed includes the subject initial and number (from Vol. I of the UG Curriculum), e.g., FM 14.1
2. Name of activity, e.g., seminar on bioethics or bedside clinic in treatment of poisoning (if the institution has numbered each activity, the number may be entered)
3. Date the activity gets completed
4. Attempt at activity by learner—indicate if:
   a. First attempt (or) only attempt
   b. Repeat (R) of a previously done activity
   c. Remedial activity (Re) based on the determination by the faculty
5. Rating—use one of three grades:
   a. Below expectations (B)
   b. Meets expectations (M)
   c. Exceeds expectations (E)
6. Decision of faculty
   a. C: activity is completed, therefore closed and can be certified, if needed
   b. R: activity needs to be repeated without any further intervention
   c. Re: activity needs remedial action (usually done after repetition did not lead to satisfactory completion)
7. Initial (Signature) of faculty indicating the completion or other determination
8. Initial (Signature) of the learner if feedback has been received.

The assessor will sign the assessment form with appropriate feedback to the students. The students also must put his/her signature on the form of assessment after understanding the different aspects mentioned in the feedback provided by the assessor.

General Instructions

1. This manual is part of the logbook and a record of the academic activities of the designated student, who would be responsible for maintaining his/her manual.
2. The student is responsible for getting the entries in the manual verified by the Faculty In-Charge regularly.
3. Entries in the manual will reflect the activities undertaken in the department and have to be scrutinized by the head of the department.
4. The manual is a record of various activities by the student like:
   - Overall participation and performance
   - Attendance
   - Participation in sessions
   - Record of completion of pre-determined activities
   - Acquisition of selected competencies
5. The manual is the record of work done by the candidate in that department/specialty and should be verified by the college before submitting the application of the students for the university examination.
6. The manual remains in the possession of the student and has to be submitted in the department during the 7th semester practical examination for final assessment. However, the "Logbook" includes other activities as detailed under Sections 2, 3 and 4 will be assessed by the assessor periodically.
7. The competencies included in the manual ensures achievement of all mandatory elements in the course and will be signed at the end of the course by the assessor(s) and Head of the Department. In the appraisal form, a student must achieve the level of 'competent' along with other criteria stipulated by the MCI, to be eligible for appearing in Final Part I MBBS University Examination in the subject of Forensic Medicine and Toxicology.

Instructions to the Students for Practical Classes

1. The students should attend all the practicals and should maintain punctuality.
2. They should wear a clean white laboratory coat with a name tag during the practicals.
3. They should maintain silence and discipline during all practical works. Mobile phones should be kept in the switched off mode.
4. They should bring the practical files during their classes and should carry one ballpen, ruler, hand lens and colored pencils.
5. They should listen carefully to the instructions given by the teacher for a particular practical and should come well prepared for the same. In case of any doubt, they should ask the relevant questions.
6. They should write the practicals accordingly, make entries in the index of the practical file and get it signed by the teacher.
7. If a student has not finished a practical, he/she should complete it on his/her own and get the practical file checked from the concerned teacher on the next working day.
8. They shall be marked as absent in the subsequent class, if found to be with incomplete work.
9. They should avoid spillage, and cleanliness at the site of work should be maintained at all times.
10. Diagrams should be made by using pencils and proper color code for various structures.

General Instructions for the Examination of a Patient and Filling up of Proformas

1. The examination of a patient should take place in adequate light, after making the patient comfortable, maintaining privacy, in the presence of a female attendant (if a male doctor examining a female patient) and after taking informed consent for the examination and intervention.
2. In all the certificates issued by the medical practitioner, the names of the doctor and the patient (examinee) should be complete and in capitals (block letters) and not initials. The address should be properly written with the house number (apartment/unit number), street, nearby landmark, city/town, state, pin code and mobile number mentioned, wherever possible.

Contents

UNIT 3: Injury — 53

UNIT 4: Sexual Offences — 89

UNIT 5: Death Certification — 126

UNIT 6: Postmortem Examination — 135

SECTION 2—Self-Directed Learning (SDL)

SECTION 3—Attitude, Ethics and Communication (AETCOM)

Phase II—MBBS 267

Phase III—Part I MBBS 283

SECTION 4—Simulation Based Teaching (Skill Lab), Vertical Integration and Seminar

SKILLS

1

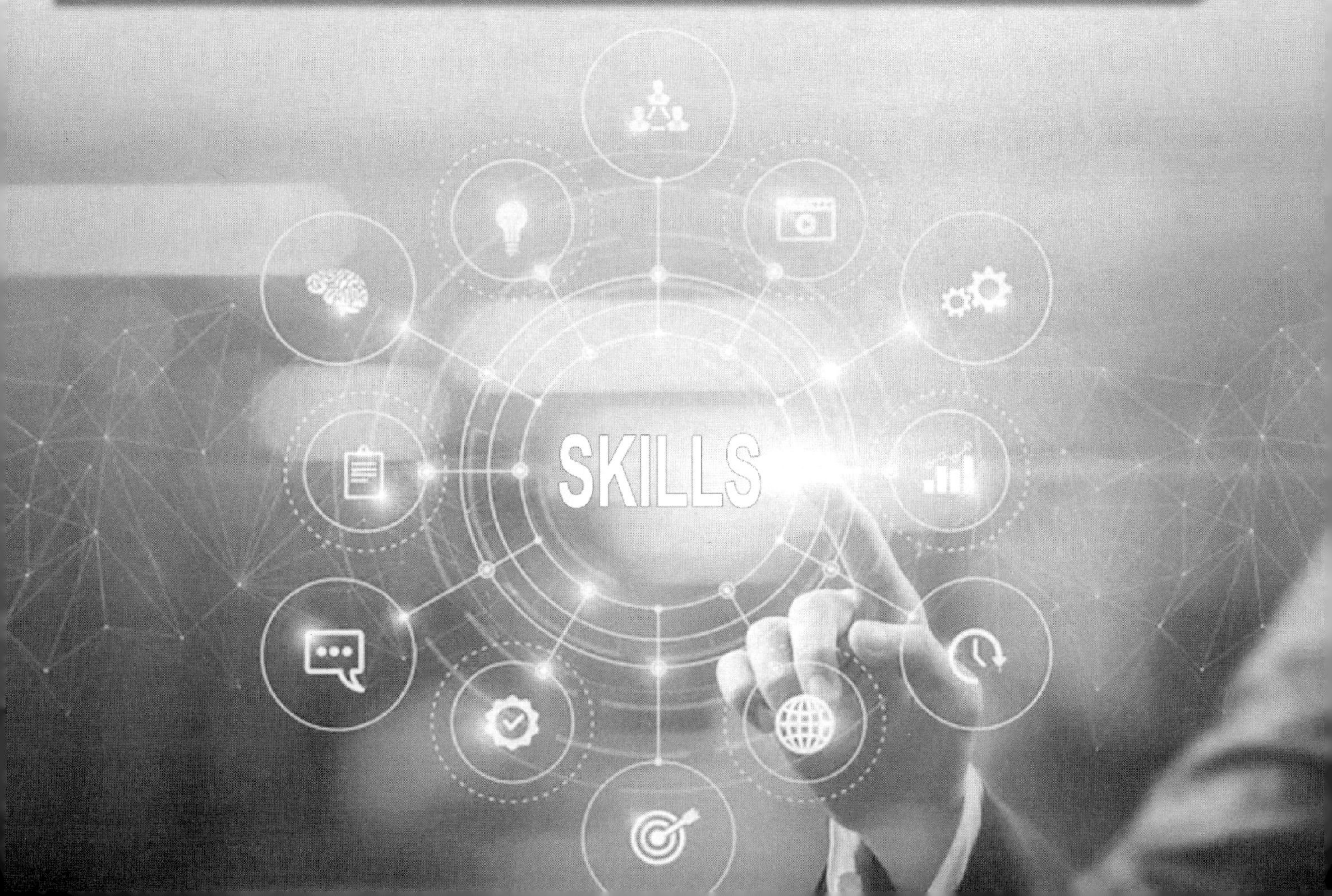

Record Sheet of Skills

(As per the Revised CBME Guidelines 2024)

Sl. No.	Page No.	Competency Addressed	Name of the Activity	Date Completed (dd-mm-yy)	Attempt at activity First or Only (F) Repeat (R) Remedial (Re)	Rating Below (B) Expectations Meet (M) Expectations OR Numerical Score	Decision of faculty Completed (C) Repeat (R) Remedial (Re)	Initial of faculty	Feedback Received Initial of learner
1.	65-76	**FM 14.1:** Examine and prepare medico-legal report of an injured person with different etiologies in a simulated/supervised environment.							
2.	79-80	**FM 14.2:** Demonstrate the correct technique of clinical examination in a suspected case of poisoning and prepare medico-legal report in a simulated/supervised environment.							
3.	81-83, 146-148	**FM 14.3:** Assist and demonstrate the proper technique in collecting, preserving and dispatch of the exhibits in a suspected case of poisoning, along with clinical examination.							
4.	33-41	**FM 14.4:** Conduct and prepare report of estimation of age of a person for medico-legal and other purposes and prepare medico-legal report in a simulated/supervised environment.							
5.	126-134	**FM 14.5:** Examine and prepare Medical Certificate of Cause of Death (MCCD) in a simulated/supervised environment.							
6.	154-226	**FM 14.6:** Conduct and prepare postmortem examination report of varied etiologies (at least 15) in a simulated/supervised environment.							

Sl. No.	Page No.	Competency Addressed	Name of the Activity	Date Completed (dd-mm-yy)	Attempt at activity First or Only (F) Repeat (R) Remedial (Re)	Rating Below (B) Expectations Meet (M) Expectations OR Numerical Score	Decision of faculty Completed (C) Repeat (R) Remedial (Re)	Initial of faculty	Feedback Received Initial of learner
7.	52	**FM 14.7:** Demonstrate the correct technique to perform and identify ABO and Rh blood group of a person.							
8.	22-32	**FM 14.8:** Demonstrate examination of and present an opinion after examination of skeletal remains in a simulated/ supervised environment							
9.	232-239	**FM 14.9:** Demonstrate ability to identify and prepare medico-legal inference from specimens obtained from various types of injuries, e.g., contusion, abrasion, laceration, firearm wounds, burns, head injury and fracture of bone.							
10.	53-56, 77-78	**FM 14.10:** To identify and describe weapons of medico-legal importance which are commonly used, e.g., lathi, knife, kripan, axe, gandasa, gupti, farsha, dagger, bhalla, razor and stick. Able to prepare report of the weapons brought by police and to give opinion regarding injuries present on the person as described in injury report/ postmortem (PM) report so as to connect weapon with the injuries. (Prepare injury report/ PM report to connect the weapon with the injuries).							
11.	57	**FM 14.11:** Describe the contents and structure of bullet and cartridges used and to provide medico-legal interpretation from these.							
12.	149-153	**FM 14.12:** To estimate the age of fetus by postmortem examination.							

Sl. No.	Page No.	Competency Addressed	Name of the Activity	Date Completed (dd-mm-yy)	Attempt at activity First or Only (F) Repeat (R) Remedial (Re)	Rating Below (B) Expectations Meet (M) Expectations OR Numerical Score	Decision of faculty Completed (C) Repeat (R) Remedial (Re)	Initial of faculty	Feedback Received Initial of learner
13.	105-112, 121-125	**FM 14.13:** To examine and prepare report of an alleged accused person in cases of various sexual offences in a simulated/supervised environment. Demonstrate an understanding of framing the preservation and dispatch of trace evidences in such cases. Describe and discuss personal opinions and their impact on such examinations and the need for objectivity/neutrality to avoid prejudice influencing the case.							
14.	92-105, 113-120, 121-125	**FM 14.14:** To examine and prepare medico-legal report on an alleged victim/survivor of various sexual offences in a simulated/supervised environment. Demonstrate an understanding of framing the opinion, preservation and dispatch of trace evidences in such cases. Describe and discuss sympathetic/empathetic examination and interview of victims/survivors of sexual assault, including presence of trusted adult figure (person) in cases of minor victims/survivors.							
15.	84-88	**FM 14.15:** To examine and prepare medico-legal report of drunk person in a simulated/supervised environment.							
16.	240-248	**FM 14.16:** To identify and draw medico-legal inference from common poisons, e.g., dhatura, castor, cannabis, opium, aconite, copper sulphate, pesticides compounds, marking nut, oleander, nux vomica, abrus seeds, snakes, capsicum, calotropis, lead compounds and tobacco.							

Sl. No.	Page No.	Competency Addressed	Name of the Activity	Date Completed (dd-mm-yy)	Attempt at activity First or Only (F) Repeat (R) Remedial (Re)	Rating Below (B) Expectations Meet (M) Expectations OR Numerical Score	Decision of faculty Completed (C) Repeat (R) Remedial (Re)	Initial of faculty	Feedback Received Initial of learner
17.	13-14	**FM 14.17:** To examine and prepare medico-legal report of a person in police, judicial custody or referred by court of law and violation of human rights as requirement of NHRC, who has been brought for medical examination.							
18.	17-19	**FM 14.18:** To record and certify dying declaration in a simulated/supervised environment.							
19.	42	**FM 14.19:** To collect, preserve, seal and dispatch exhibits for DNA-finger printing.							
20.	20-21	**FM 14.20:** To give expert medical/medico-legal evidence in court of law.							
21.	10-12, 126-134	**FM 1.9:** Describe the importance of documents in medical practice in regard to: Documents for issuance of death certificate, Documents of Medical Certificate of Cause of Death (MCCD) (Form 4A).							
22.	126-134	**FM 1.11:** Write the correct cause of death certificate as per ICD-11 document.							
23.	43-51	**FM 12.5:** Demonstrate the professionalism while preparing reports in medico-legal situations, interpretation of findings of biological or trace evidences.							
24.	249-254	To identify and prepare medico-legal inference from histopathological slides of myocardial infarction, pneumonitis, tuberculosis, brain infarct, liver cirrhosis, brain hemorrhage, bone fracture, pulmonary edema, brain edema, soot particles, diatoms, wound healing and bronchopneumonia.							

Certifiable Procedural Skills

(As per the Revised CBME Guidelines, 2024)

Sl. No.	Page No.	Name of Activity	Date Completed dd-mm-yy	Attempt at activity First or Only (F) Repeat (R) Remedial (Re)	Rating Below (B) Expectations Meet (M) Expectations OR Numerical Score	Decision of faculty Completed (C) Repeat (R) Remedial (Re)	Initial of faculty and date	Feedback Received Initial of learner
1.	58-76	Examine and prepare medico-legal report of an injured person with different etiologies in a simulated/ supervised environment.						
2.	126-134	Examine and prepare Medical Certificate of Cause of Death (MCCD) in a simulated/ supervised environment. Write a correct Medical Certificate of Cause of Death (MCCD) certificate as per ICD 11 document.						
3.	135-226	Conduct and prepare postmortem examination report of varied etiologies (at least 15) in a simulated/ supervised environment.						
4.	105-112	To examine and prepare report of an alleged accused person in cases of various sexual offences in a simulated/supervised environment.						
5.	92-104	To examine and prepare medico-legal report on an alleged victim/survivor of various sexual offences in a simulated/ supervised environment.						

Postmortem Examination Reports

Sl. No.	Date	Cause of death	Page No.	Signature of Teacher
1.				
2.				
3.				
4.				
5.				
6.				
7.				
8.				
9.				
10.				
11.				
12.				
13.				
14.				
15.				

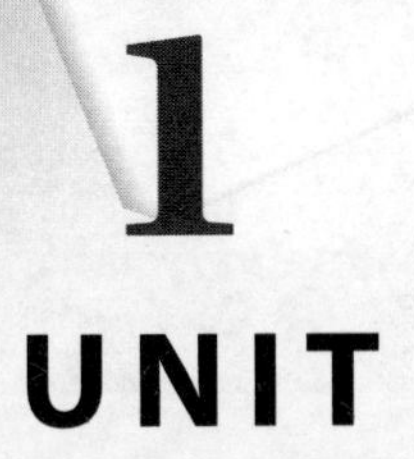

1
UNIT

Medical Jurisprudence and Legal Procedure

Write drug therapy for Amit Banerjee, 45-year-old male, residing at Quarter No. 1567, Lodi Road Colony, New Delhi, who is found to be hypertensive during routine medical examination. His height is 174 cm and weight is 82 kg and BP is 160/118 mm Hg. No other abnormality found.

____ (Doctor's name)

_________________________________ (Qualification)

_________________________________ (State Medical Council Registration Number)

____ (Full address)

___________________________ (Clinic telephone No.) _______________________ (E-mail ID)

____

Prescription serial No. ___________________   Date _________________

Patient's name ____________________________________ Age ___________ Gender ______________

Contact details ____ (Complete address of patient)

Mobile No. ___________________ E-mail ID ___________________

Diagnosis ___________________________________   Weight _______________

    (for pediatric patients)

R̟X

1. _________________________________ (Generic name of medicine in capital letters only)
   (Strength, dosage form, dosage instruction, duration and total quantity)

2. _________________________________ (–do–)

3. _________________________________ (–do–)

    (   )

    Doctor's signature and date

    Seal

DISPENSED

Date: _________   Name of pharmacist: ___________________

Address of pharmacist/medical store ____

EX. 1.2: SICKNESS CERTIFICATE

FM 1.9: Describe the importance of documentation in medical practice in regard to issuance of sickness certificate.

Prepare a sickness certificate for 2 weeks for Jatin Pandey, 24-year-old male, residing at Quarter No. 657/A, Defense Colony, New Delhi, who is suffering for pneumonia which was diagnosed clinically and confirmed by laboratory tests. He has a small black mole 0.1 × 0.1 cm on the tip of his nose and a linear white scar mark measuring 1.5 × 0.5 cm on his right cheek.

Report No.___________________

Signature or thumb impression of the patient

(To be filled in by the applicant in the presence of the Government Medical Practitioner)

Identification marks:

1. _______________________________________

2. _______________________________________

I, Dr ____ after careful examination hereby certify that

Mr/Ms ___________________________________ S/D/W of _______________________________________

aged about _________ years, residing at ____ and whose

signature/thumb impression is verified above is suffering from ______________________________________.

I consider that a period of absence from duty of ____ with effect from

____ is absolutely necessary for the restoration of his/her health.

(   )

Place __________________

Date __________________

Signature and Seal of Medical Practitioner

Registration No. _______________________

(State Medical Council of .... State)

Note: The nature and probable duration of the illness should also be specified. This certificate must be accompanied by a brief resume of the case giving the nature of the illness, its symptoms, causes and duration.

EX. 1.3: FITNESS CERTIFICATE

FM 1.9: Describe the importance of documentation in medical practice in regard to issuance of fitness certificate.

Draft a fitness certificate for Jatin Pandey, 24-year-old male, residing at Quarter No. 657/A, Defense Colony, New Delhi, who has recovered from pneumonia and to report on duty, for whom you issued a sickness certificate 2 weeks back. He has a small black mole 0.1 × 0.1 cm on the tip of his nose and a linear white scar mark measuring 1.5 × 0.5 cm on his right cheek.

Report No._____________________

Signature or thumb impression of the patient

(To be filled in by the applicant in the presence of the Government Medical Practitioner)

Identification marks:

1. ____

2. ____

This is to certify that I, Dr ____ have carefully examined

Mr/Ms _______________________________ S/W/D of _______________________________,

aged about _______________________ years, resident of _______________________________ and whose

signature/thumb impression is verified above and found that he/she has completely recovered from his/her illness.

He/She is now fit to resume duties in Government/private service with effect from _______________________________.

I also certify that before arriving at this decision, I have examined the original medical certificate and statement of the case on which leave was granted or extended and have taken them into consideration in arriving at my decision.

(   )

Place _________________   Signature and Seal of Medical Practitioner

Date _________________   Registration No. _______________________

(State Medical Council of ……….…..… State)

Note: This certificate must be accompanied by a brief resume of the case giving the nature of the illness, its symptoms, causes and duration.

EX. 1.4: CERTIFICATE OF MEDICAL FITNESS
(To be deposited at the time of joining and obtained only from Gazetted Government Medical Practitioner)

FM 1.9: Describe the importance of documentation in medical practice in regard to issuance of fitness certificate.

Draft a medical fitness certificate for job recruitment for Bimal Dass, 21-year-old male, height 176 cm and weight 75 kg. He has a black mole of size 0.1 × 0.1 cm on his right side forehead just above the eyebrow and a birthmark measuring 1.5 × 1.0 cm on his left thumb on its outer aspect.

Report No.________________________

Name ____

Father's name ____

Blood group______________   Height_________ cm   Weight _________ kg

Chest ____

Heart and lungs ____

Vision   Left _______________________________   Right__________________________

Color vision ____

Hearing ____

Hernia/Hydrocele/Piles ____

Any other disease diagnosed in past ____

Allergies, if any ____

List of prescribed medication, if any:

1. ________________________________

2. ________________________________

3. ________________________________

Any other remarks: ____

I certify that I have carefully examined Mr/Ms ____

son/daughter of Mr _________________________________ who has signed in my presence.

He/she has no physical disease and is medically fit.

Signature of the candidate

Place ________________

Date ________________

____
Signature of Medical Practitioner

Name, Designation and Seal

EX. 1.5: CERTIFICATE OF EXAMINATION OF AN ARRESTED PERSON

FM 14.17: To examine and prepare medico-legal report of a person in police, judicial custody or referred by court of law and violation of human rights as requirement of NHRC, who has been brought for medical examination.

Draft a certificate for Sayed Hussain, 40-year-old male, residing at 456/35-C, Mohalla Shiv Puri, Janakpuri, New Delhi who was arrested by the police for alleged murder of his business partner and brought for examination. He has a black mole of 0.2 × 0.1 cm on his right ear and a linear white scar mark measuring 8.5 × 2.5 cm on his left forearm on its outer aspect.

Report No. _________________   Date _____________

As per requisition from _______________________________ dated ___________________, physical examination of

Mr/Ms _________________________________ S/D/W of _________________________________,

residing at ____, involved in FIR No. _________________

of police station _______________________ was done on ________________ at _____________ AM/PM.

<table>
<tr><td>Consent</td><td>Identification marks</td></tr>
<tr><td>I have voluntary agreed for the medical examination and investigations. I have been explained that it was necessary for diagnosis and treatment of the disease from which I may be suffering. This has been explained in ________________ language which I understand.

Signature/Thumb impression of the examinee</td><td>1. _______________________________

____

2. _______________________________

_______________________________</td></tr>
</table>

History (related to illness/injury, if any) ____

Physical Examination

A. General: Build and nourishment: Poor/Moderate/Obese

   Height ________ cm   Weight ________ kg   Pulse ________ /min

   Blood pressure___________ mm Hg   Pallor: Present/Absent

   Physical deformity, if any ____

   Others, if any: ____

B. Systemic examination

   1. Central nervous system ____

   2. Cardiovascular system ____

   3. Respiratory system ____

   4. Gastrointestinal system ____

C. Injuries, if any (use body diagrams) ____

D. Investigations, if any ____

Opinion

There is no evidence of any clinically identifiable illness.

There are no injuries on the person/injuries on the person which could be caused as alleged.*

Suggestions, if any ____

Place ____________   Signature of Medical Practitioner

Date__________   Name, Designation and Seal

*Strike off which is not applicable

EX. 1.6: INFORMATION TO HEALTH AUTHORITIES REGARDING NOTIFIABLE DISEASES
(Privileged Communications)

Tularam Gaitonde, a 65-year-old man who came from London 5 days back is admitted in your hospital with the symptoms of COVID-19 (high fever, cough, breathlessness, sore throat, etc.). You have already collected the nasal and throat swab samples and sent them for testing, the RT-PCR test has come positive. He has been kept in an isolation ward. Inform your local health authority regarding the same.

CASE DEFINITION ______________________________

Clinical information

Physician name–Last name	First name	Telephone number

Patient information

Last name	First name	Middle name

Father's/Guardian's name _______________________________________

Age_______ years

Gender ☐ Male ☐ Female ☐ Other_______

Pregnant ☐ Yes ☐ No ☐ Unknown

If Yes, Estimated delivery date (____ /____ /________)

Address ____

County of residence ________________

Country of birth, if not Indian born ________________

Date of arrival in India (mm/dd/yyyy) ________________________

Telephone number ____________ Mobile number ☐☐☐☐☐☐☐☐☐☐

E-mail ____________________________

Occupation (Describe/Specify) _______________________________

Primary language _______________________

Race (*Tick '✓'*)

☐ Indian ☐ White ☐ African-American/Black ☐ American Indian

☐ Japanese ☐ Korean ☐ Chinese ☐ Other: ____________

Signs and symptoms

Symptomatic? ☐ Yes ☐ No ☐ Unknown	*Onset Date (mm/dd/yyyy)*	*Date First Sought Medical Care (mm/dd/yyyy)*

Signs/Symptoms (Specify) ______________________________

____

____

____

Past medical history ____

Hospitalization

Did patient visit emergency room for illness? ☐ Yes ☐ No ☐ Unknown	Was patient hospitalized? ☐ Yes ☐ No ☐ Unknown	If Yes, how many total hospital nights?

Hospitalization – Details ____
____

Outcome

Outcome? ☐ Survived ☐ Died ☐ Unknown	If survived, Survived as of _______________ (mm/dd/yyyy)	Date of death (mm/dd/yyyy)

Laboratory information

Specimen Type 1 ☐ Serum ☐ CSF ☐ Other _______________	Type of test	Specimen type 2 ☐ Serum ☐ CSF ☐ Other _______________	Type of test

Laboratory results summary – Other ____

Epidemiologic information

Travel history

Did patient travel outside of county of residence during the incubation period? ☐ Yes ☐ No ☐ Unknown	Has the patient traveled outside India during the incubation period? ☐ Yes ☐ No ☐ Unknown

If yes for either of these questions, specify all locations and dates below.

Travel history–details

Location (city, county, state, country)	Date travel started (mm/dd/yyyy)	Date travel ended (mm/dd/yyyy)

Exposures/risk factors ____

Reporting agency

Investigator name	Local health jurisdiction	Telephone number	Date (mm/dd/yyyy)

First Reported By

☐ Clinician ☐ Laboratory ☐ Other (specify): _______________

State use only

Case classification ☐ Confirmed ☐ Probable ☐ Suspected ☐ Not a case ☐ Need additional information

EX. 1.7: RECORDING OF DYING DECLARATION BY A MEDICAL PRACTITIONER

FM 14.18: To record and certify dying declaration in a simulated/supervised environment.

Chandanika Swain, a 25-year-old female, married last year, is admitted in your hospital with alleged history of being burnt by her parents-in-law and her husband who sprinkled kerosene oil on the clothes and set her on fire, and bolted the door of her room from outside. The neighbors on hearing her screaming and shouting, rescued her and brought to the hospital in critical condition. She has 95% burns. Record her dying declaration since there is no time to call the Magistrate. (Note: Take the declaration from the patient only. Do not make any cutting/overwriting or change the pen. Do not take thumb impression in case of a 100% burn case).

I, Dr ____ S/D/W of ____,

working as ____________________________________, residing at ____

in presence of witnesses (1) ________________________________ S/D/W of ________________________________

residing at ________________________________ and witness (2) ________________________________

S/D/W of ________________________________ residing at ________________________________ shall record the

dying declaration of Mr/Ms ________________________________ aged about ____________ years,

S/D/W of ________________________________ married/unmarried, occupation ____________________

residing at ____ at ____________ AM/PM, on

____________ (date), at ________________________________ (place) in the word by word

order as narrated by the declarant.

Certification of Compos Mentis

Questions that may be asked:
a. What is your name?
b. What is the year/season/date/month?
c. Whether it is morning/evening/night?
d. Where do you live?
e. Where do you think you are?
f. Are you married? What is the name of your eldest sibling?
g. What is you education?

I have thoroughly examined his/her level of consciousness, orientation of time and space, memory and other mental faculties and I hereby certify that the declarant is in possession of a sound mind to deliver his dying declaration.

I, Dr ____, have come to record your dying declaration.

Will you be able to answer my questions?   Yes/No

Dying Declaration

Before recording this dying declaration, I have examined the declarant and found that his/her condition is critical and he/she may die any time hereafter, in spite of the lifesaving treatment being given to him/her. The words of the declarant as said by him/her are: _______________________

____

____

____

____

In order to clarify the points as revealed by above and in continuation to this, I asked the following questions to which the declarant gave the answers, which are recorded in that sequence:

i.   Why were you brought to the hospital? (describe the incident in detail since beginning)

____

____

____

____

____

ii. At what time the incident took place?

____

iii. How, by whom, under what circumstances and at which place, did you sustain injury?

____

____

____

iv. What is the reason behind this incident?

____

____

v.   Did you have any past enemy?

____

vi. Who were present at the time of the incident?

____

____

vii. Anything else that you want to mention about the incident?

____

____

viii. Can you sign/put thumb impression?

____

The above recorded dying declaration is correct as per my dictation which I am signing after reading that bear my signature/thumb impression (should be translated into declarant's mother tongue by a translator).

I, Dr ____ certify that the above declaration was recorded by me.

I also certify that the declarant Mr/Ms ____ maintained

his/her sound state of mind throughout the dictation of his/her declaration. The recording ended at ______________ AM/PM on ____________________.

	__________________________
	Signature of Medical Practitioner
	(Name, Designation and Seal)

Signature/Thumb impression of declarant

Place ________________

Date ________________

Signature of the translator ___________________________________

Name and address ____

Recorded and signed in our presence

1. Signature, Name and Address of first witness ____

2. Signature, Name and Address of second witness ____

EX. 1.8: EXPERT EVIDENCE IN THE COURT OF LAW

FM 14.20: To give expert medical/medico-legal evidence in court of law.

You have examined a 19-year-old female with alleged history of rape. In the medico-legal report, you mentioned 'a tear at the 5-6 o'clock position which was fresh. It extended right through the hymen extending just inside the vagina. Around the area was a further area of skin loss. The area was red, macerated and extremely sore. The whole lesion was about 2.0 × 1.0 cm'. You have been summoned in this case. Write down the steps to be followed by you so as to provide expert evidence in the court of law. How would you prepare yourself for the case? What are the possible alternative interpretations of the injury? What is your opinion regarding consensual sex and the above mentioned injury?

Identification

EX. 2.1: EXAMINATION OF SKELETAL REMAINS

FM 14.8: Demonstrate examination of and present an opinion after examination of skeletal remains in a simulated/supervised environment.

A primary school student while playing in the mountains discovered a skeletonized femur, and reported this to his mother. During a search of the vicinity, the right femur, right tibia, pelvis and skull (depressed fracture present in right parietal area) along with mandible (2 mandibular and 7 maxillary teeth were present, rest missing) were discovered. The police sent it to you to determine whether they belong to the same person (since the sites of discovery differed) and whether identity and cause of death could be established. Draft a report for the same.

Department of Forensic Medicine and Toxicology

Report No. _______________   Date _______________

Requisition from ____ Dated _______________

Brought by _____________________________________ P.C. No. _______________________ P.S. _________

Examination Findings

A. Description [List of bone(s) received]

☐ Complete skeleton   ☐ Partial skeleton   ☐ Fragmentary remains   ☐ Only skull

B. Condition of skeleton

☐ Cracking   ☐ Brittle   ☐ Breaks   ☐ Cut marks   ☐ Gnaw marks

☐ Exfoliation   ☐ Warping   ☐ Insect damage   ☐ Soil adhering   ☐ Staining

C. Origin of the bone (whether the bones are human or not?)

a. Anatomical characteristics ____

b. Microscopic examination ____

c. Analysis of bone ash ____

d. Precipitin test ____

D. Whether they belong to one or more individuals?

    a. Number, side and size of the bones ________________________________

    ____

    ____

    b. Age and sex ____

    c. Morphological similarities ____

    ____

    d. Use of shortwave UV light ____

    ____

    e. X-ray comparison of trabecular pattern ______________________________

    ____

    f. Neutron activation analysis ____

    ____

E. The stature of the individual to whom the bones belonged.

Multiplication factor or regression analysis. ______________________________

____

____

F. The race of the individual to whom the bones belonged.

Indices and racial peculiarities ____

____

____

G. The sex of the individual to whom the bones belonged.

    a. General characteristics ____

    ____

    b. Specific changes in the individual bone ______________________________

    ____

    c. Examination of the soft parts, if available ____________________________

    ____

H. The age of the individual to whom the bones belonged.

    a. Dental status, if skull or mandible is available _______________________

    ____

    ____

    b. Ossification data ____

    ____

    ____

    c. Secondary changes in the bones like closure of skull sutures, bony joint surfaces, etc. _____________

    ____

    ____

I.   Whether the bones have been cut, sawn, gnawed by animals or burnt? ________________________

____

____

J.   Any other feature(s) that may help in identification of the individual.

    a.   Congenital abnormalities or deformities ______________________________________

    b.   Acquired peculiarities – injuries, fractures, etc. ______________________________

    c.   Determination of the blood group from the marrow/tooth pulp __________________

    d.   Radiological examination. ____

Opinion

i.   From the above findings, I am of the opinion that the bone(s) belong to ________________

origin, of ______________________ sex and aged about ____________________________ .

ii.   Cause of death

    a.   Any injuries/fracture ____

    b.   Foreign body (bullet, pellets or any piece of weapon) ______________________

    c   Chemical analysis for poisoning ______________________________________

    d.   Neutron activation analysis ____

iii. Time since death

    a.   State of soft tissue, if available ______________________________________

    b.   Changes due to putrefaction ____

    c.   Stages of healing in case of fracture ____________________________________

____

Signature of Medical Officer
Name, Designation and Seal

____

Received Report No. ____________________, bundle of bones, packed and sealed along with the sample seal.

Name ________________________________ P.C. No. ________________ P.S. ________________

____

Signature and Date

EX. 2.1: EXAMINATION OF SKELETAL REMAINS

Report No. _______________

Fill in skeletal elements present and record notes alongside.

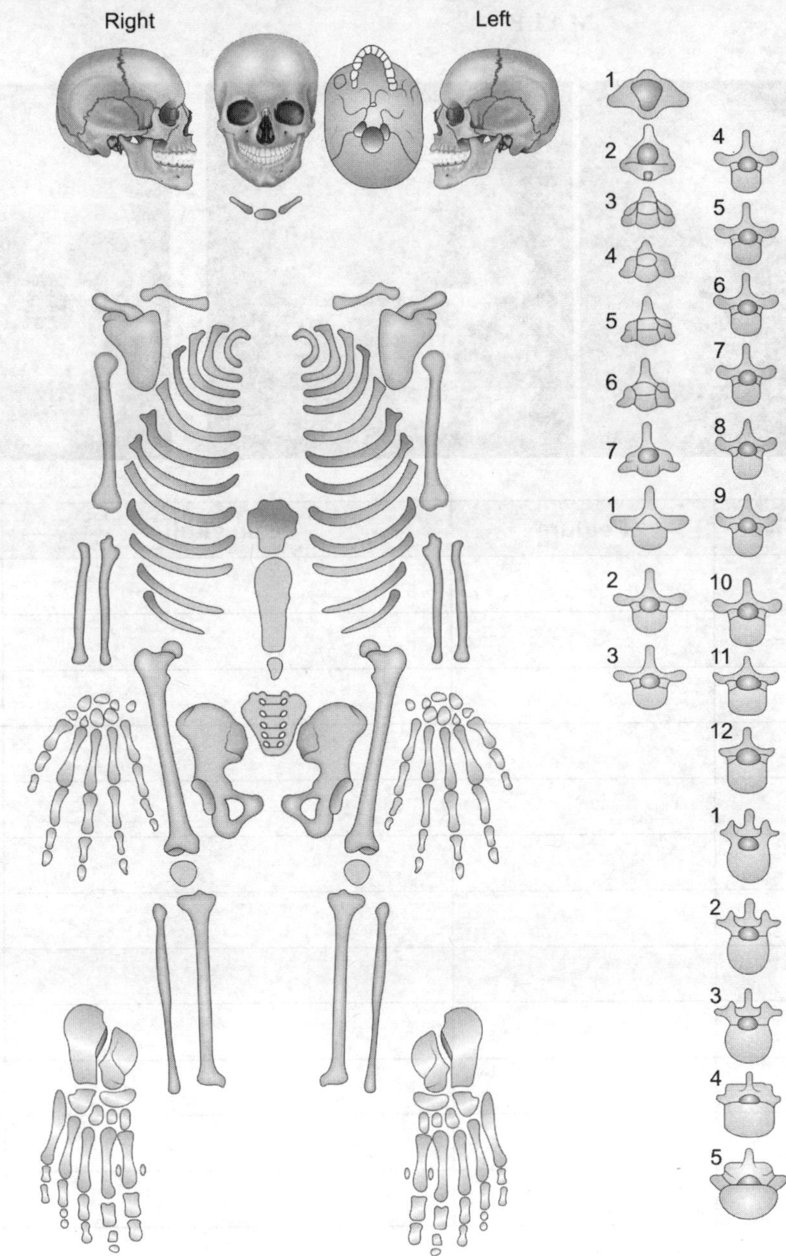

Additional observations:

EX. 2.1A: DETERMINATION OF SEX FROM SKELETAL REMAINS (Skull)

MALE

FEMALE

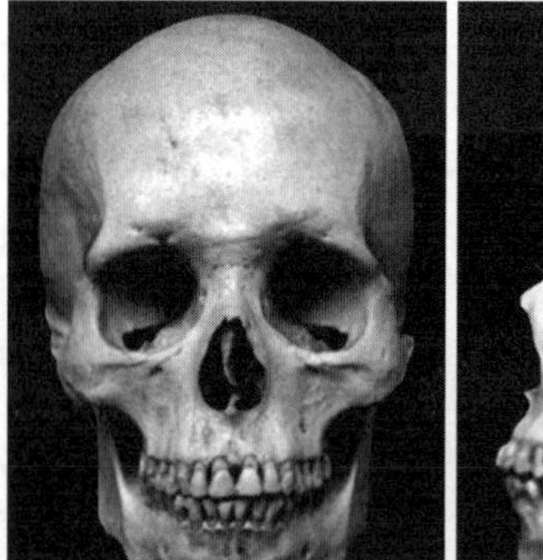
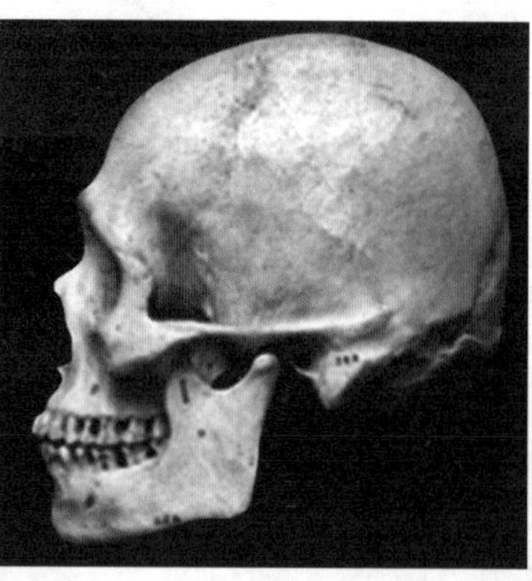
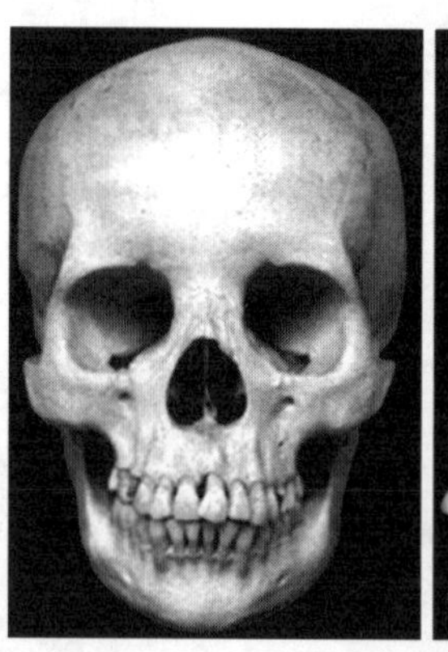
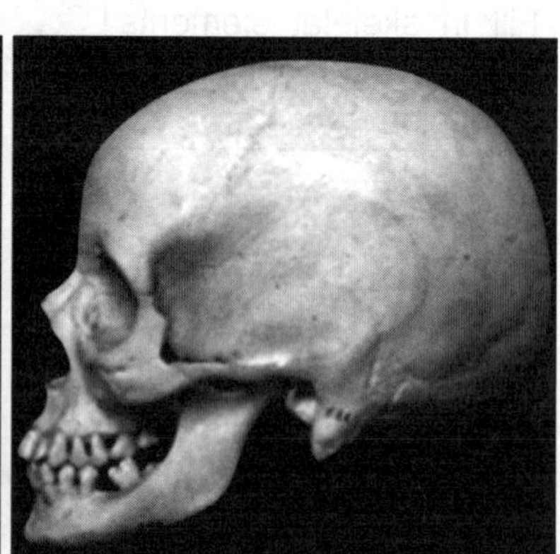

Sl. No.	Feature	Male skull	Female skull

EX. 2.1B: DETERMINATION OF SEX FROM SKELETAL REMAINS (Mandible)

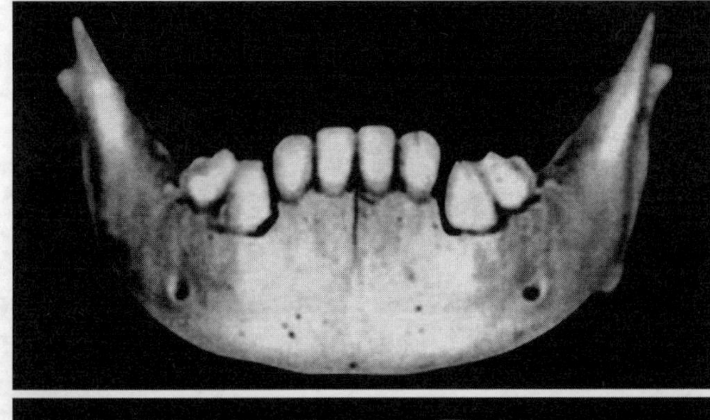
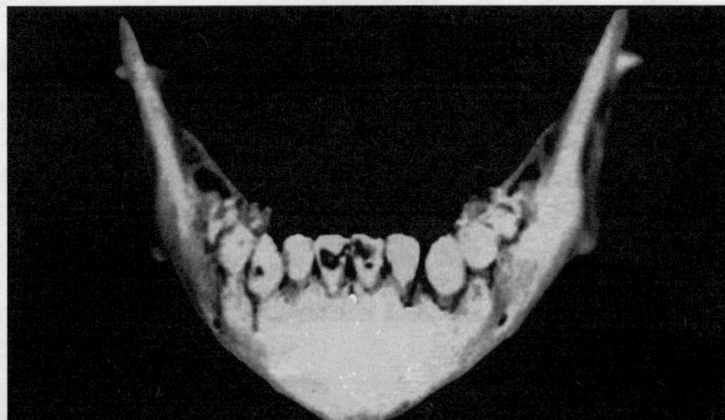
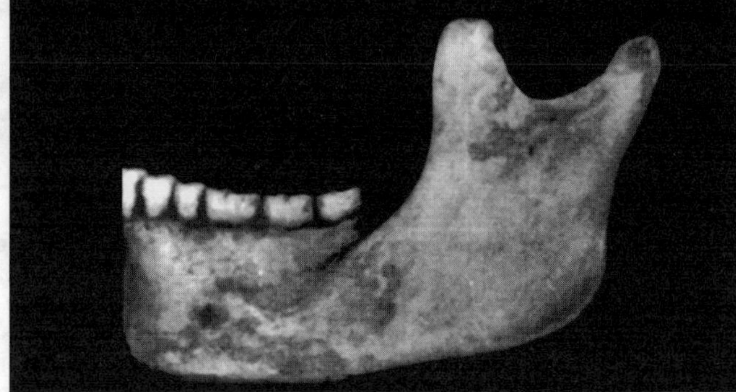
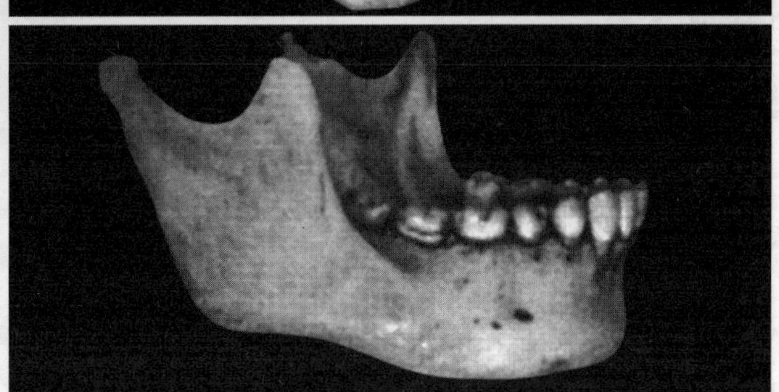

Sl. No.	Feature	Male mandible	Female mandible

EX. 2.1C: DETERMINATION OF SEX FROM SKELETAL REMAINS (Pelvis)

MALE

FEMALE

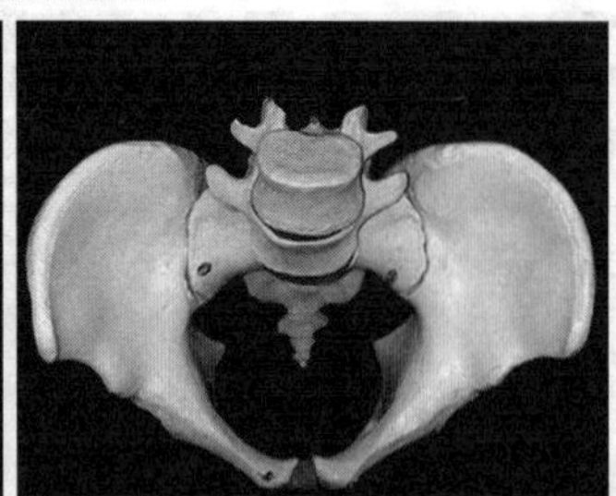 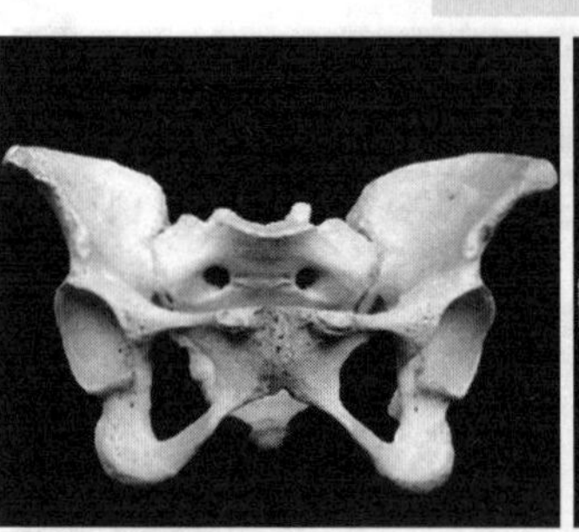 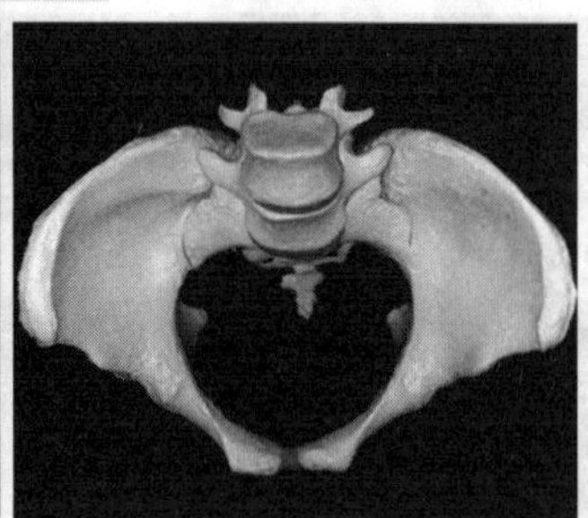

Sl. No.	Feature	Male pelvis	Female pelvis

EX. 2.1D: DETERMINATION OF SEX FROM SKELETAL REMAINS (Sacrum)

MALE

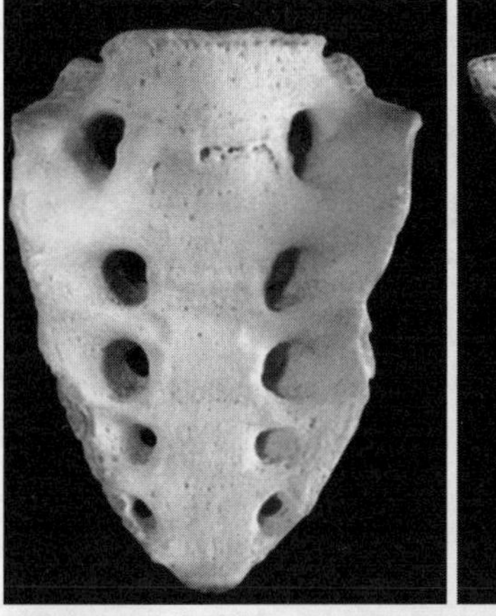
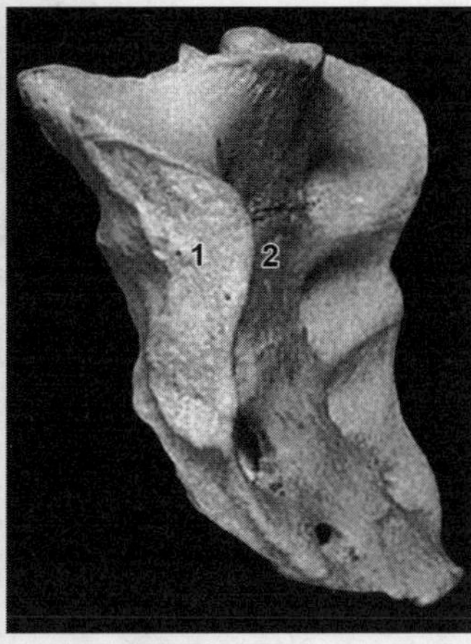

FEMALE

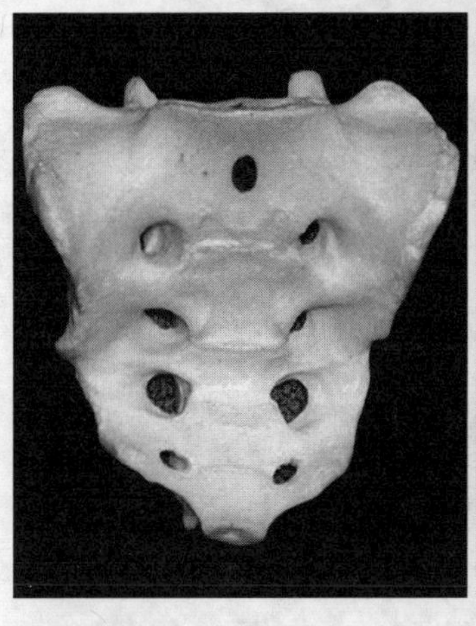
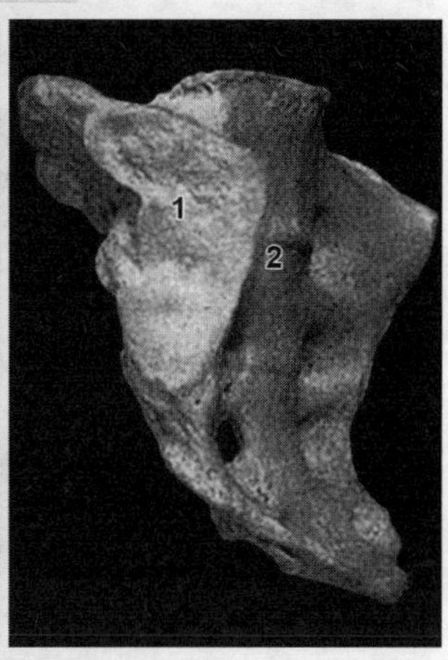

Sl. No.	Feature	Male sacrum	Female sacrum

EX. 2.1E: ESTIMATION OF AGE FROM ERUPTION OF TEETH

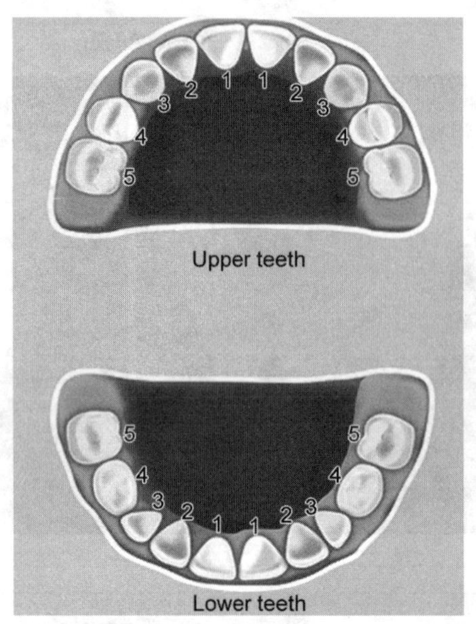

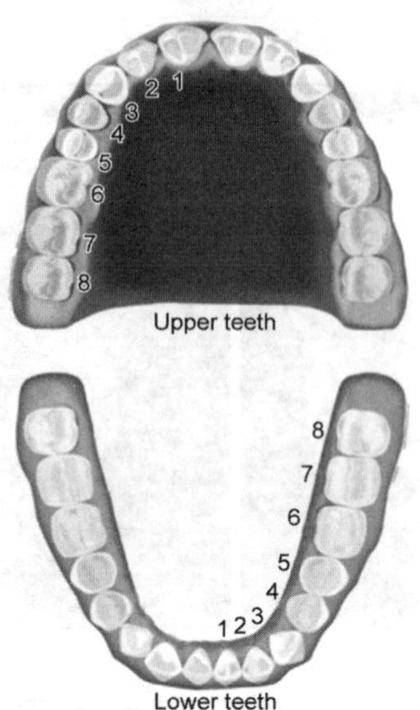

Eruption of Temporary Teeth

Teeth	Age of eruption
Central incisors Lower Upper	
Lateral incisors Upper Lower	
First molars	
Canines	
Second molars	

Eruption of Permanent Teeth

Teeth	Age of eruption
First molars	
Central incisors	
Lateral incisors	
First premolars	
Second premolars	
Canines	
Second molars	
Third molars	

EX. 2.1F: STUDY OF MANDIBLES IN DIFFERENT AGE GROUPS

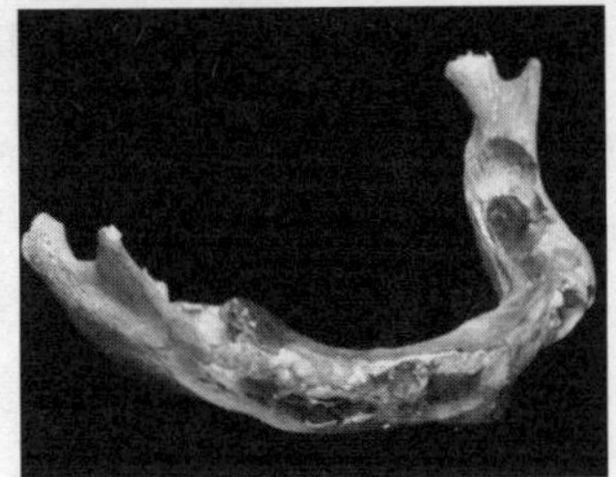

Infancy

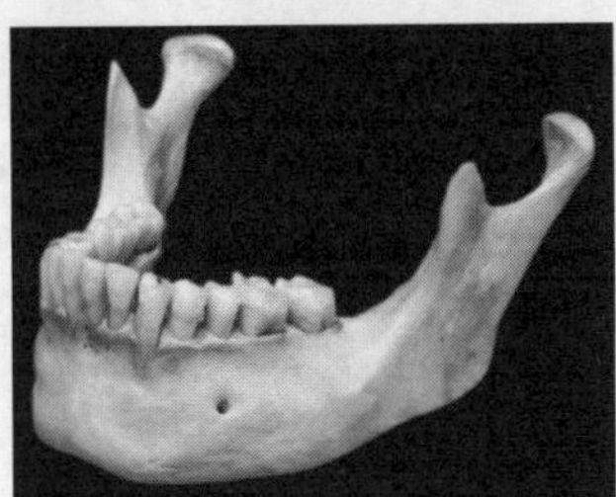

Adult

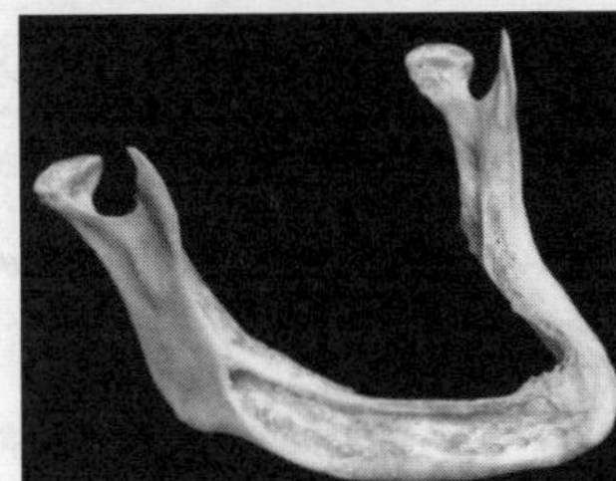

Old age

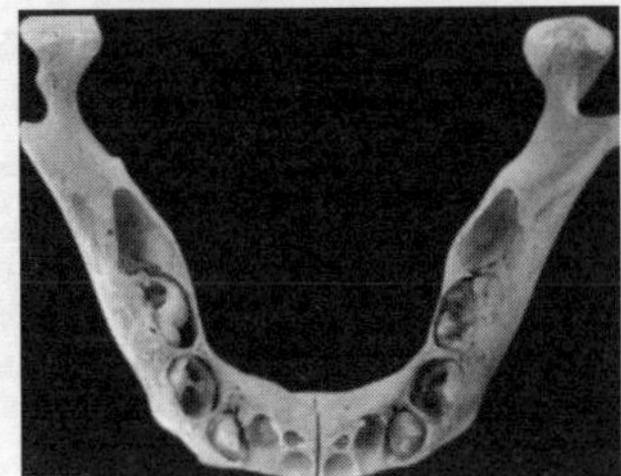

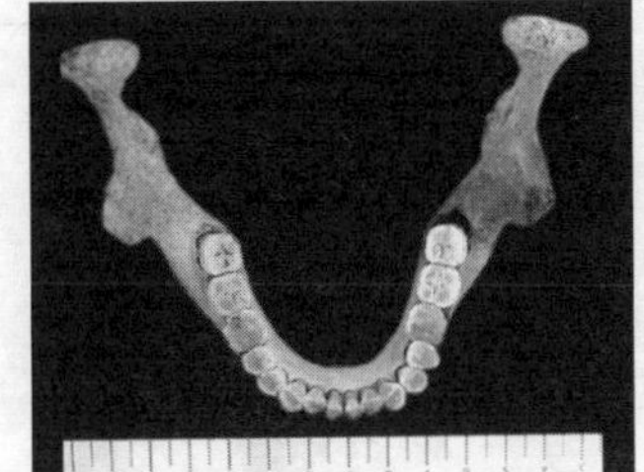

Feature	Infancy	Adult	Old age

EX. 2.1G: ESTIMATION OF STATURE FROM LONG BONES

You have been provided with the following long bones—femur, tibia, fibula, humerus, radius, ulna and clavicle. Find the stature using osteometric board.

A. **Femur:** *Stature: Length of the bone × Multiplication factor*
   Stature = L × M.F.
   (M.F. factor 3.6–3.8)

   The height of the individual is between _______________________ and _______________________ cm.

B. **Tibia and fibula**
   Stature = L × M.F.
   (M.F. factor 4.8–4.4)

   The height of the individual is between _______________________ and _______________________ cm.

C. **Humerus**
   Stature = L × M.F.
   (M.F. factor 5.30–5.0)

   The height of the individual is between _______________________ and _______________________ cm.

D. **Radius**
   Stature = L × M.F.
   (M.F. factor 6.7–6.9)

   The height of the individual is between _______________________ and _______________________ cm.

E. **Ulna**
   Stature = L × M.F.
   (M.F. factor 6.0–6.3)

   The height of the individual is between _______________________ and _______________________ cm.

F. **Clavicle**
   Stature = L × M.F.
   (M.F. factor 11.1)

   The height of the individual is about _______________________ cm.

EX. 2.2: EXAMINATION FOR AGE ESTIMATION IN LIVING PERSONS

FM 14.4: Conduct and prepare report of estimation of age of a person for medico-legal and other purposes and prepare medico-legal report in a simulated/supervised environment.

A male individual Dasarath Manjhi, son of Jiten Manjhi was brought by the police for age estimation. He was found working in a chemical factory. He claims to be 19 years old but the police booked the owner for illegal underage employment and stated his age as 14 years. He is a resident of Madhepura, Bihar. He has no birth certificate or school leaving certificate and is illiterate. Prepare a report for the same.

Department of Forensic Medicine and Toxicology

____

Report No. _____________________________   Date and Time of examination _________________________

Requisition from _______________________________Vide letter No. ____________________ Dated ________________

Name ________________________________ S/D/W of ____

Address ____

Gender ____________________________ Occupation ______________________________ Marital status ________________

Age as alleged by:

a.   Individual to be examined _______________________ years

b.   Police or person accompanying ________________ years

Brought by _____________________________ P.C. No. ____________________________ P.S. ______________________

Identification marks:

1.   ____

2.   ____

Informed Consent

I, ____ hereby voluntarily agree to the following: (*Tick '√' that applies*)

☐ Medical examination and examination of genitals and also examination of other secondary sexual characters for the purpose of age estimation.

☐ Radiological and dental examination for the purpose of age estimation.

☐ Photography for the purpose of evidence, if required.

☐ The report may be used for legal evidence, clinical audit, research and academic purposes.

☐ Inform the police and provide them the copy of this examination.*

☐ I have also been informed that I can refuse the whole or part of the examination and also refuse information to be given to the police. In this event, I will be responsible for any problem arising in the process of investigation and court trial.* I have been further informed that this refusal will not have any impact on the quality of treatment provided.

☐ The findings of the examination may go against me.

☐ All this has been explained to me in _________________________ language which I can understand.

Strike out in case examination is done under the provisions of Sec. 53 CrPC

____

____

Signature and name of the witness

Signature/Thumb impression _________________

Name _________________________________

Signature and name of the person examined or guardian (when the person is unable to give consent due to insanity or is < 12 years)

Female nurse/attendant in presence of whom examination is conducted (if applicable)	Signature _________________________ Name _________________________

General Physical Examination

Height _________ cm   Weight _____________ kg   Pulse __________ /min   B.P. __________ mm Hg

Built: Poor/average/well

Secondary Sexual Characters

Male	Female
Beard/Moustaches: Absent/downy/sparse/black/bushy	Breast development: Not developed/developing/well developed (Tanner stage _________________)
Pubic hair: Absent/downy/sparse/black/bushy (Tanner stage _________________)	Pubic hair: Absent/downy/sparse/black/bushy (Tanner stage _________________)
Axillary hair: Absent/downy/sparse/black/bushy	Axillary hair: Absent/downy/sparse/black/bushy
Voice: Masculine/Feminine (Deep/soft)	Menarche:
Adams apple: Prominent/not prominent	Last menstrual period:
Genitals: Scrotal/testicular/penile development (Tanner stage _________________)	Genitals:

Other Features

Acne _________________________

Wrinkles on face/skin _________________________

Other features, if any: ____

Eyes (Arcus senilis, cataract) _________________________

Dental Examination

Total number of teeth _________________ Temporary _____________ Permanent _________________

Type of dentition: Primary/Mixed/Permanent

Space behind 2nd permanent molar _____________________

Dentition

	18	17	16	15	14	13	12	11	21	22	23	24	25	26	27	28	
R																	L
	48	47	46	45	44	43	42	41	31	32	33	34	35	36	37	38	

P: Permanent   T: Temporary

Y: Erupted but missing   X: Not erupted

Radiological examination (For appearance and fusion of centers of ossification)

Sl. No.	Part X-rayed	Observations	Inference

Orthopantomograph (OPG) findings: ____

____

____

OPINION

After performing general physical, dental and radiological examination, I am of the opinion that age of the subject

is above _______________ years and below _______________ years of age.

(_____________________)

Place _________________   Signature of Medical Officer

Date _________________   Name, Designation and Seal

____

Received Report No. ___________________________________

Name ____ P.C. No. _______________ P.S. _______________

Signature and date

Requisition for Radiological Examination for Estimation of Age
Department of Forensic Medicine and Toxicology

Ref. No _________________ Date _________________

To

The Professor/Medical Officer I/C

Department of Radiology

____

Subject: Estimation of age of ____

Dear Sir/Madam,

Ref. Requisition from ____ dated _________________

I request that radiographs of the subject may be taken as indicated below.

Sl. No.	Region	View

The subject bears the following identification marks:

1. ____

2. ____

I request you that the X-ray plates may be sent to me at the earliest.

Yours faithfully

____

Place _________________

Signature of Medical Officer

Date _________________

Name, Designation and Seal

EX. 2.2A: DETERMINATION OF AGE FROM X-RAYS

Determine the age of the male individuals from the given X-rays.

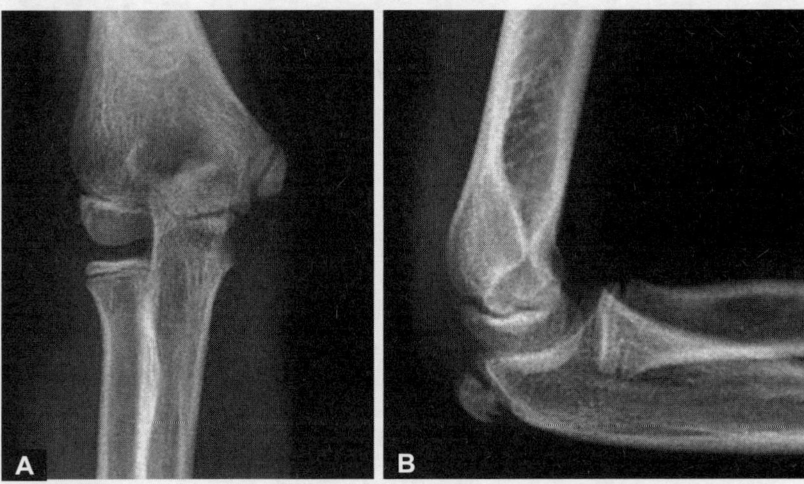
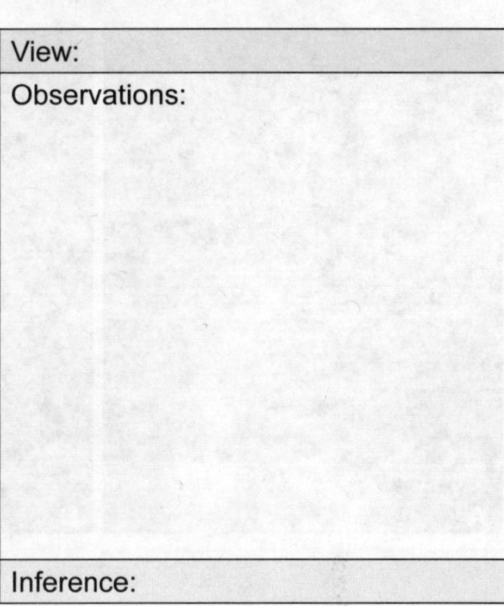

View:
Observations:
Inference:

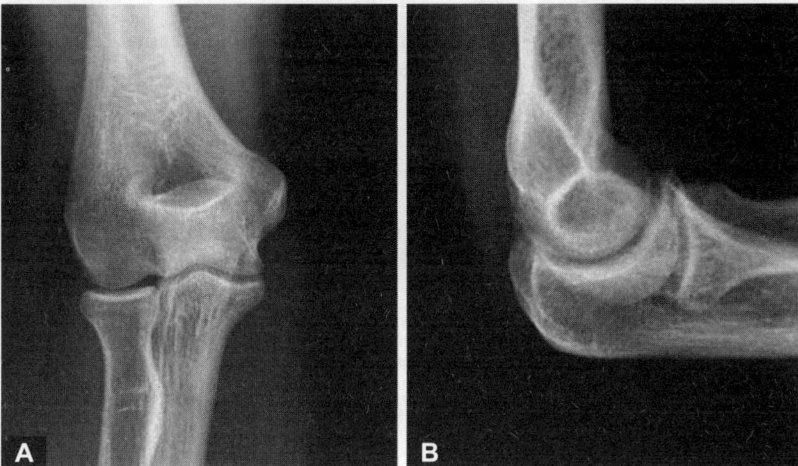
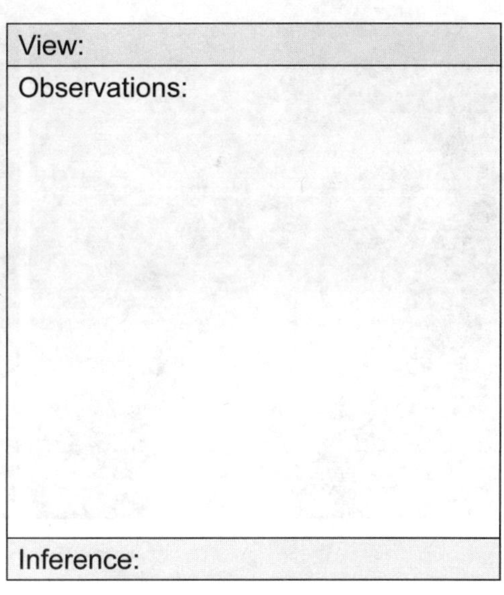

View:
Observations:
Inference:

EX. 2.2B: DETERMINATION OF AGE FROM X-RAYS

Determine the age of the male individuals from the given X-rays.

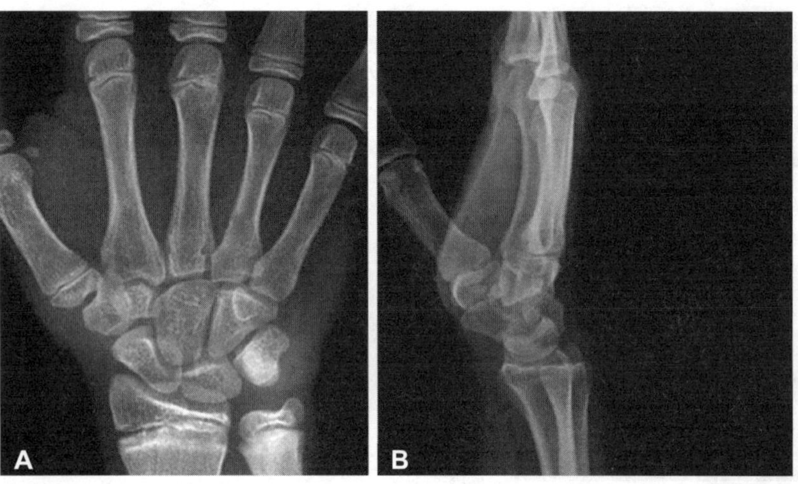

View:
Observations:
Inference:

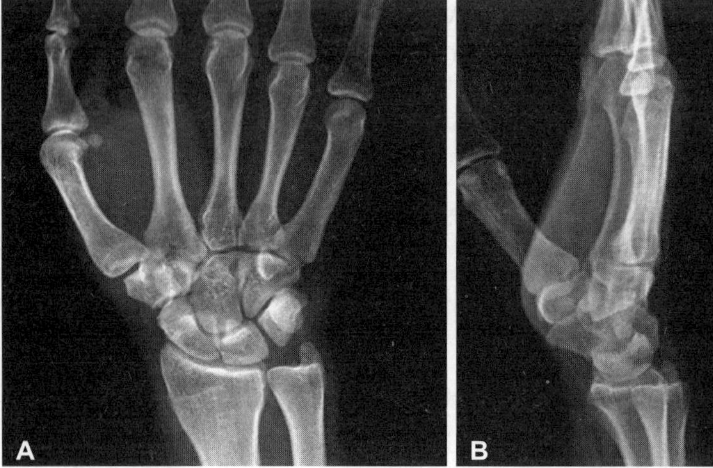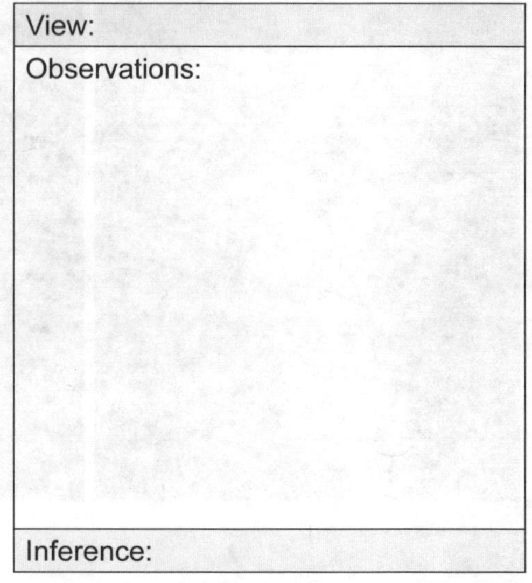

View:
Observations:
Inference:

EX. 2.2C: DETERMINATION OF AGE FROM X-RAYS

Determine the age of the male individuals from the given X-rays.

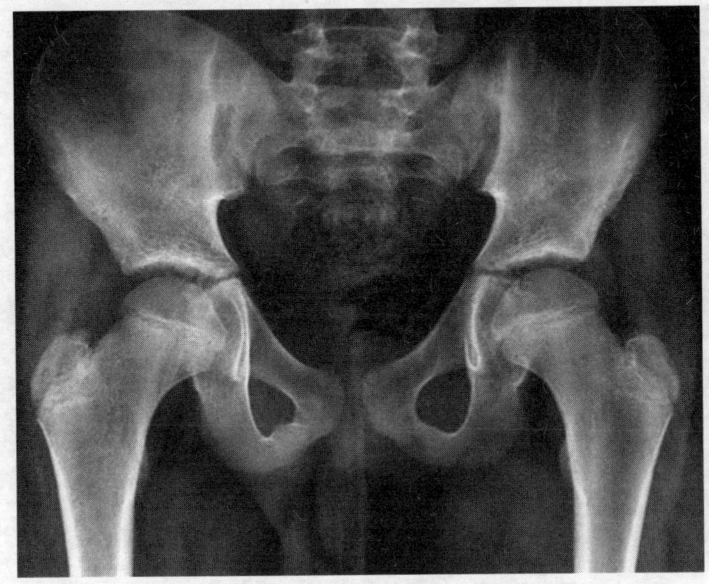

View:

Observations:

Inference:

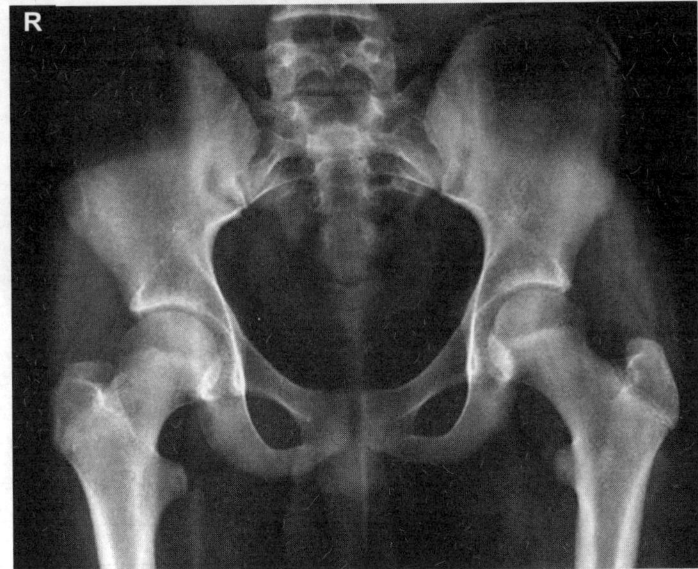

View:

Observations:

Inference:

EX. 2.2D: DETERMINATION OF AGE FROM X-RAYS

Determine the age of the male individuals from the given X-rays.

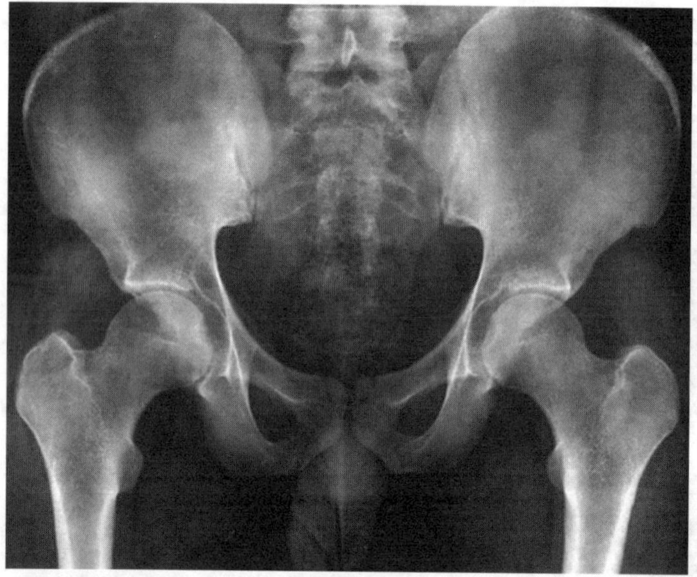

View:
Observations:
Inference:

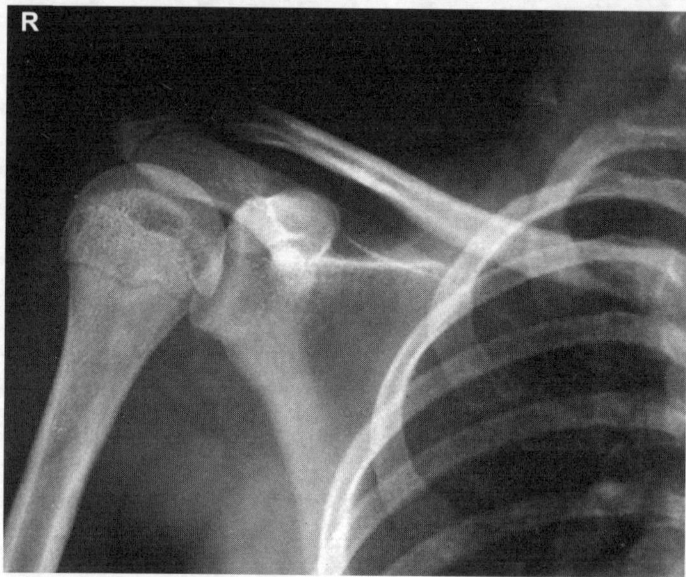

View:
Observations:
Inference:

EX. 2.2E: FINGERPRINT CARD

Applicant	Leave Blank	Last name	First name	Middle name	Leave Blank

Signature of person fingerprinted	Date of birth Month Day Year

Residence of person fingerprinted	Citizenship	Sex	Race	Ht.	Wt.	Eyes	Hair	Place of birth

Date	Signature of official taking fingerprints	Aadhaar Card No.	Leave Blank
Employer and address		Driving License No.	Class ______________________________
		Employee Code	Ref.______________________________
Reason fingerprinted		Passport No.	
		Miscellaneous No.	

1. R. Thumb	2. R. Index	3. R. Middle	4. R. Ring	5. R. Little

6. L. Thumb	7. L. Index	8. L. Middle	9. L. Ring	10. L. Little

Left four fingers taken simultaneously	L. Thumb	R. Thumb	Right four fingers taken simultaneously

EX. 2.3: BIOLOGICAL SPECIMEN COLLECTION FORM FOR DNA TESTING

FM 14.19: To collect, preserve, seal and dispatch exhibits for DNA-Finger printing.

Case Particulars

Name ____

Father/Guardian's name _______________________________________

Gender _______________   Age _______years _______months

Address ____

Medical history ____

____

Genetic abnormalities, if any _________________________________

Blood transfusion, if any, in past 3 months ____________________

Organ transplantation, if any _________________________________

Affix a passport size signed photograph of the donor attested by medical officer in presence of I.O. or a gazetted officer.

Sample Collected for Case Examination

Case no. _______________ Date: ______________ P.S. ____________ U/S ______________

Description of sample *(Tick '✓')*

☐ Blood in EDTA   ☐ Blood in FTA card

☐ Oral swab   ☐ Vaginal swab   ☐ ______________

Date of collection ___________________ Collected by ___________________

Purpose for conducting test ____

____

Seal impression:
(Wax covered with cellotape)

____
Signature of Medical Practitioner
Name, Designation, and Seal

Declaration of the Donor/Guardian

I, ______________________________________ S/D/W/under guardianship of Mr/Ms______________________

hereby declare that the biological sample(s) (______________________) thus being collected for DNA profiling is with my consent and is mine/is of my child. I/he/she did not receive any blood transfusion within past 3 months.

Signature ______________________

Name ______________________

Left thumb impression   Right thumb impression   Date ______________________

Collection of biological sample should be preferably in presence of two witnesses.

Witness 1

Signature ____________________

Name _______________________

Date _______________________

Witness 2

Signature ____________________

Name _______________________

Date _______________________

EX. 2.4: EXAMINATION OF HAIR

FM 12.5: Demonstrate the professionalism while preparing reports in medico-legal situations, interpretation of findings of biological or trace evidences.

A. Structure of hair ____

____

Hair or fiber ____

____

B. Source of hair

    a. Human or animal hair _______________________________________

        Medullary index _______________________________________

____

    b. Racial differences _______________________________________

____

    c. Male or female hair _______________________________________

____

    d. Place of origin from the body _______________________________

____

C. Other information

    a. Age of the person _______________________________________

____

    b. Any alteration/disease _______________________________________

____

    c. Naturally removed or traumatic _______________________________

____

    d. Toxicological information _______________________________________

____

D. Medico-legal importance

____

____

____

____

____

Difference between Hair and Fiber

Feature	Hair	Fiber

Difference between Human Hair and Animal Hair

Feature	Human Hair	Animal Hair

EX. 2.5: EXAMINATION OF SEMINAL STAINS

FM 12.5: Demonstrate the professionalism while preparing reports in medico-legal situations, interpretation of findings of biological or trace evidences.

A. Purpose of examination ____

____

____

B. Methods of examination

    i.   Physical examination (quality, viscosity, odor, solubility, appearance): _______________

____

____

    ii. Examination under U-V light ____

____

    iii. Chemical Examination

        a. **Florence test**

           Procedure ____

____

____

           Observations ____

____

        b. **Barberio's test**

           Procedure ____

____

____

           Observations ____

____

        c. **Acid phosphatase test (Brentamine fast blue test)**

           Procedure ____

____

____

           Observations ____

____

iv. **Microscopic examination**

Procedure ____

____

____

Observations ____

____

v. **Other staining methods and noncellular semen markers**

a. Christmas tree stain ____________________________________

____

b. Acid phosphatase test (quantitative) ____________________

____

c. Prostate specific antigen (p30) __________________________

____

d. Semenogelin ____

____

vi. **Species origin** ______________________________________

____

____

vii. **Individualization of seminal stains**

a. Blood group—Secretors/Nonsecretors____________________

____

____

b. Enzyme typing ____

____

____

c. DNA profiling ____

____

____

C. **Medico-legal issues**

____

____

____

____

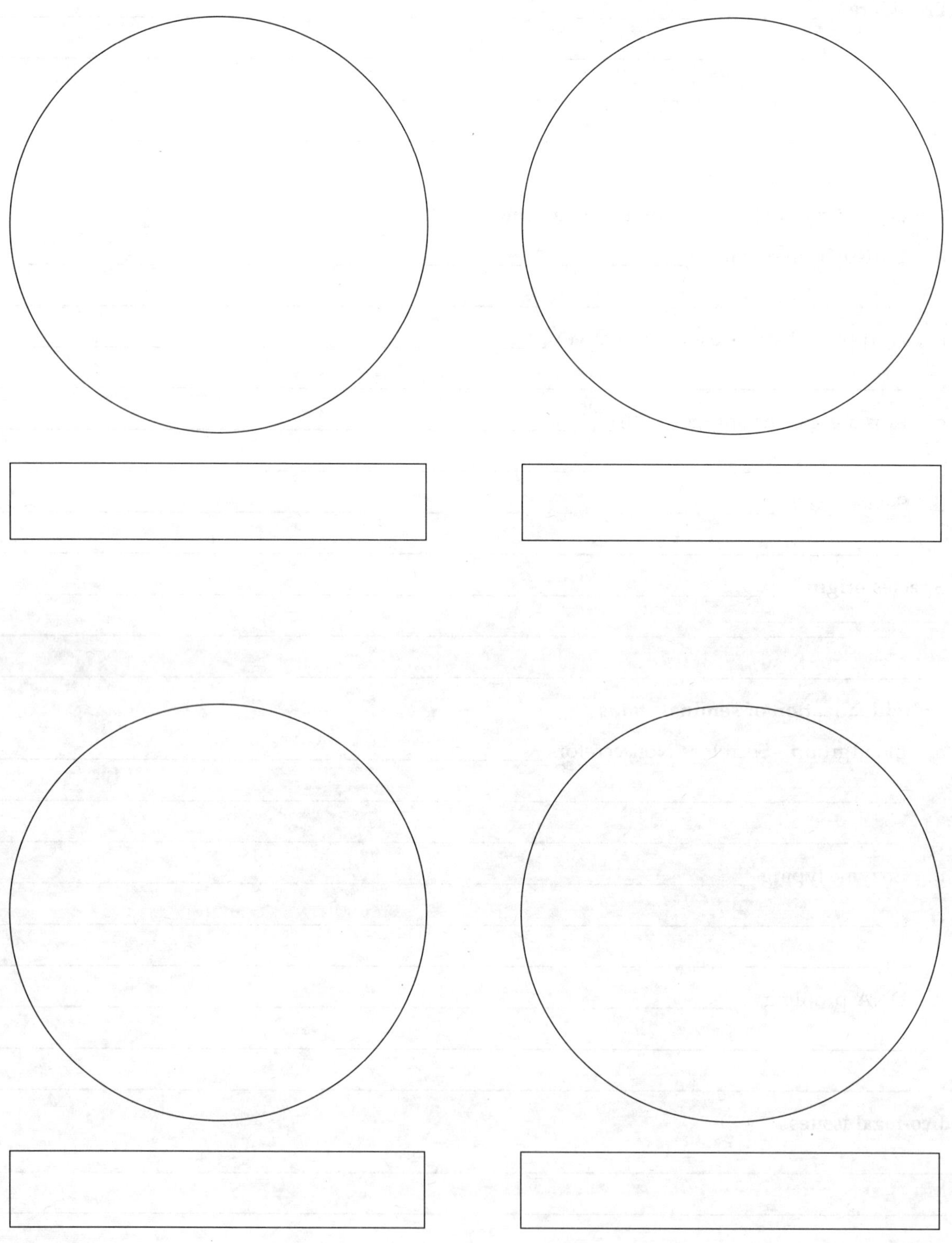

EX. 2.6: EXAMINATION OF BLOODSTAINS

FM 12.5: Demonstrate the professionalism while preparing reports in medico-legal situations, interpretation of findings of biological or trace evidences.

A. Purpose of examination ____

____

____

B. Methods of examination

    a. Physical examination ____

____

    b. Chemical examination **(Phenolphthalein test or Kastle-Meyer test)**

        Procedure____

____

____

        Observations ____

____

    c. Microscopic or Microchemical Examination

        i. **Hemochromogen crystal test (Takayama test)**

            Procedure ____

____

____

            Observations____

____

        ii. **Hemin crystal test (Teichmann's test)**

            Procedure____

____

____

            Observations____

____

    d. **Microscopic examination** (Human or animal blood)

____

____

____

____

e. **Spectroscopic examination**

____

____

____

____

f. **Biological/Serological examination**

i. Precipitin test _______________________________

____

____

____

____

ii. Blood grouping (ABO and Rh typing) _______________

____

____

____

____

C. Medico-legal issues

____

____

____

____

____

____

____

____

____

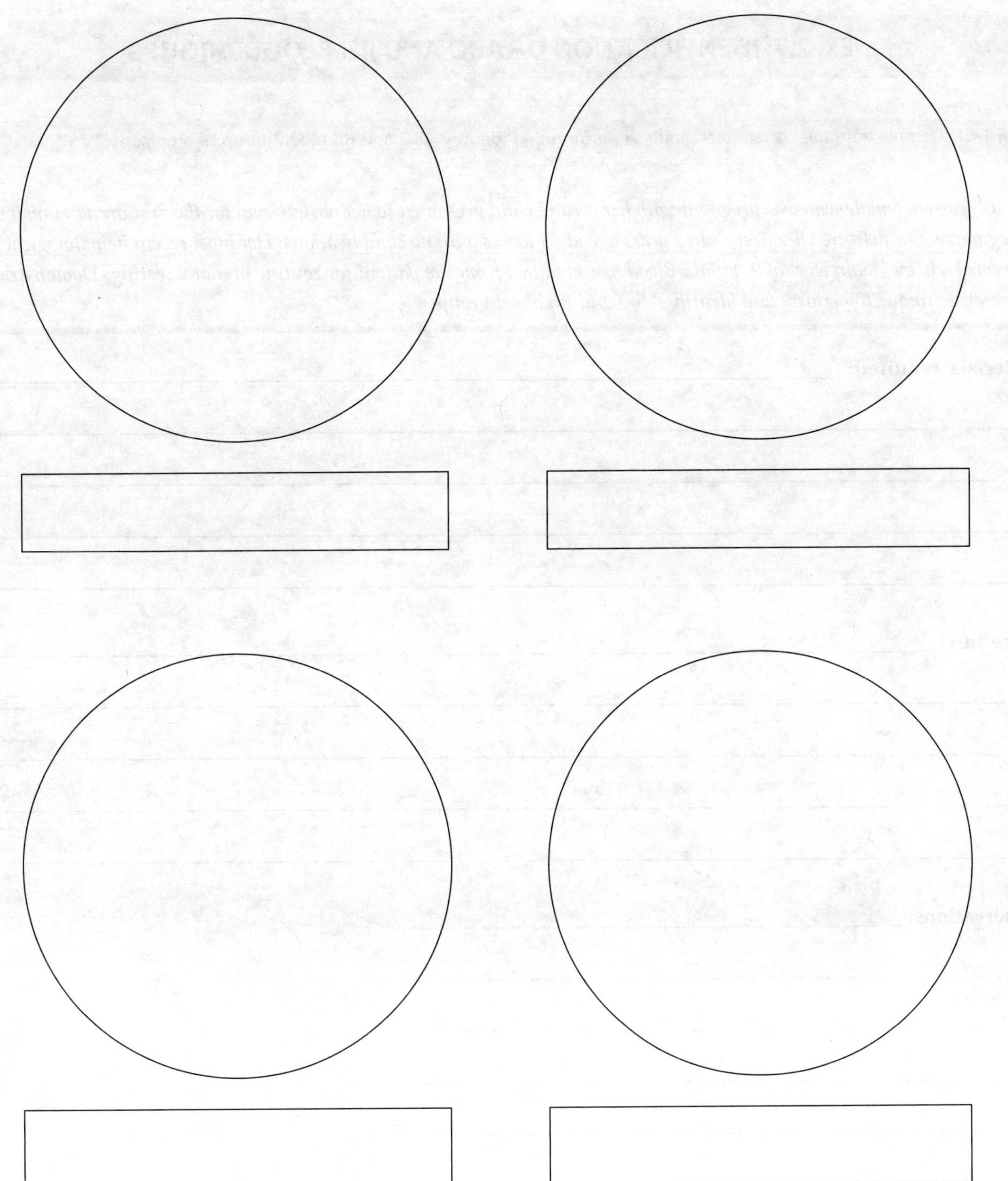

EX. 2.7: IDENTIFICATION OF ABO AND RH BLOOD GROUPS

FM 14.7: Demonstrate the correct technique to perform and identify ABO and Rh blood group of a person.

A 30-year-old female who was pregnant with her second child presented to her obstetrician for the first prenatal visit of this pregnancy. She delivered her first child 3 years ago at 39 weeks with no complications. Her most recent hematological study revealed a hemoglobin level of 9.0 g/dL. Blood was obtained from the patient for routine prenatal testing. Demonstrate the correct technique to perform and identify ABO and Rh blood group.

Materials required: ____

____

____

____

____

Procedure: ____

____

____

____

____

Observations: _______________________________________

____

____

____

Inference: ____

____

____

____

Injury

FM 14.10: To identify and describe weapons of medico-legal importance which are commonly used, e.g., lathi, knife, kirpan, axe, gandasa, gupti, farsha, dagger, bhala, razor and stick. Able to prepare report of the weapons brought by police and to give opinion regarding injuries present on the person as described in injury report/PM report so as to connect weapon with the injuries. (Prepare injury report/PM report to connect the weapon with the injuries).

Weapon	Description, injuries possible and MLI
Name:_______________	Description and type Type of injuries produced Medico-legal importance
Name:__________ Name:__________	Description and type Type of injuries produced Medico-legal importance
Name:_______________	Description and type Type of injuries produced Medico-legal importance

EX. 3.1B: EXAMINATION OF COMMON WEAPONS OF OFFENCE

Weapon	Description, injuries possible and MLI
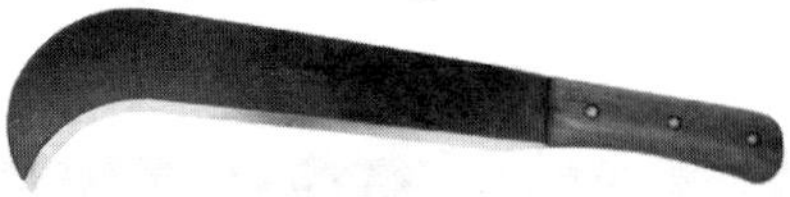 Name:________________	Description and type Type of injuries produced Medico-legal importance
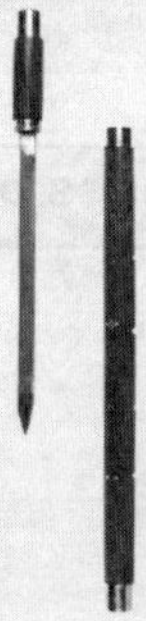 Name:________________	Description and type Type of injuries produced Medico-legal importance
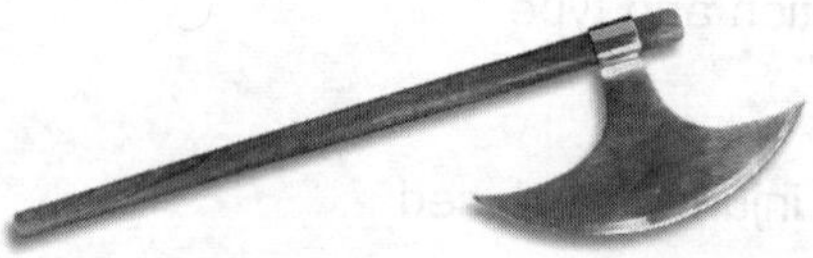 Name:________________	Description and type Type of injuries produced Medico-legal importance
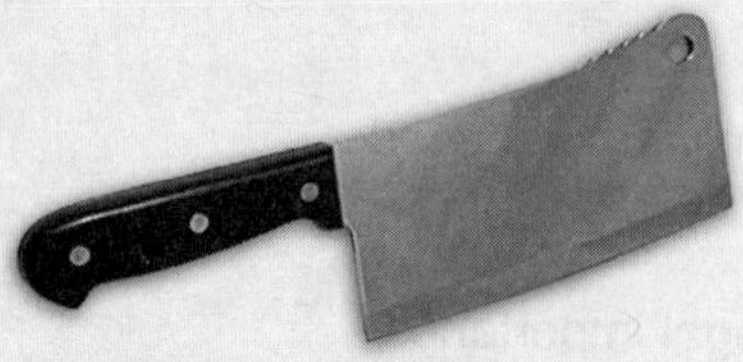 Name:________________	Description and type Type of injuries produced Medico-legal importance

EX. 3.1C: EXAMINATION OF COMMON WEAPONS OF OFFENCE

Weapon	Description, injuries possible and MLI
Name:_________________	Description and type Type of injuries produced Medico-legal importance
Name:_________________	Description and type Type of injuries produced Medico-legal importance
Name:_________________	Description and type Type of injuries produced Medico-legal importance
Name:_________________	Description and type Type of injuries produced Medico-legal importance

EX. 3.1D: EXAMINATION OF COMMON WEAPONS OF OFFENCE

Weapon	Description, injuries possible and MLI
Name:_________________	Description and type Type of injuries produced Medico-legal importance
Name:_________________	Description and type Type of injuries produced Medico-legal importance
Name:_________________	Description and type Type of injuries produced Medico-legal importance
Name:_________________	Description and type Type of injuries produced Medico-legal importance

EX. 3.2: EXAMINATION OF FIREARM CARTRIDGE

FM 14.11: Describe the contents and structure of bullet and cartridges used and to provide medico-legal interpretation from these.

Parts of Bullet

Contents:

Medico-legal significance:

Parts of Shotgun cartridge

Contents:

Medico-legal significance:

MEDICO-LEGAL REPORT/INJURY REPORT

Medico-legal case: A case of injury or ailment where the medical practitioner after history taking and clinical examination considers that investigations by law enforcement agencies are necessary to ascertain circumstances of the causation of the said injury or ailment.

Medico-legal Report

A medico-legal report (MLR) is a report on the condition of a patient, solicited for legal purposes which gives the medical expert's findings, diagnosis, prognosis and opinion. It is a structured and formal mode of communication between the doctor and the legal system.

The format should help the medical officer to give a comprehensive report that clearly separates the facts from the opinions, and provides a basis for the opinion stated.

GUIDELINES FOR WRITING A MLR

- Medico-legal injury cases should be examined without delay at anytime of the day or night.
- All details of examination of the injured person, whether admitted into hospital or treated in OPD have to be entered in a Medico-legal Register.
- This register is a confidential record and should be in safe custody of the medical officer. It has to be produced in the court of law, if asked for.
- The particulars are entered in the injury report by the medical practitioner in his/her own handwriting (at some places computerized reports are being issued).
- Cutting/overwriting should be avoided as much as possible and all corrections should be properly initialed. It should be corrected legibly by lining out with a single line, initializing with date.
- The report should be comprehensive without being unnecessarily wordy and over-inclusive.
- The report is usually addressed to the police and the lawyers who are not themselves experts in medical field. Hence, the report should be written in clear and understandable English, with as little use of technical terms and professional jargon as possible.
- Abbreviations should be avoided—write all the entries including the medical terms in a full form. Symbol '#' used to denote a fracture in medical notes should not be used in MLRs. 'Contused lacerated wound' instead of 'c.l.w' is to be written.
- During examination of a female subject by a male doctor, a nurse/female attendant MUST BE PRESENT.
- The report should always be signed by the medical practitioner to authenticate it along with date, his/her full name, designation, registration number, current employment and qualifications at appropriate place.

Date and Time of Examination

- Every MLR must include the date and time of examination.
- It is important to include the time when the examination began and ended, as this may support the contention that the examination was a complete and thorough one.

Consent

Before starting of examination, informed written consent from the patient or the legal guardian is to be taken in writing (preferably in presence of disinterested witness).

Identification Marks

- It is better to note down at least two identification marks.
- If only one identification mark is recorded, there may be a chance of loss of one mark due to any reason—scarification or amputation of that part; and during subsequent examination it may cause difficulty in identification.

The marks used for identification:

- Congenital marks—birth marks, moles, nevus, supernumerary teeth/fingers, cleft palate, etc.
- Acquired marks—scar, tattoo, deformities, malunited fractures, etc.

History

'Alleged' short history of the case is noted as stated by the patient/persons accompanying the patient. If the patient is conscious and able to speak, history of the incidence is recorded from the patient. If the patient is unconscious, history of the incidence is then taken from the persons accompanying the patient. Questions should include:

a. Date and time of infliction of injury.
b. How the injury was sustained, if assaulted, number of persons involved?
c. Whether any weapon was used, if so what type of weapon; if it was hard, blunt or sharp cutting or pointed, etc.
d. Whether any first aid/treatment was given at any place?

If serious, dying declaration is recorded as required.

General Physical Examination

- Consciousness, orientation, pulse, temperature, blood pressure, reaction of pupils to light.
- Size of the victim, i.e., stature, weight and development (in case of children/adolescents).

Examination of Injuries

A few basic items are also essential prior to examination: a hand lens, measuring scale and a torch, and the injuries are described as given in **Table 3.1**. The injuries should be highlighted in a separate body diagram too.

Table 3.1: Describing features of physical injuries.

Feature	Notes
Type	All injuries, i.e., abrasion, contusion, laceration, incised wound, etc., observed, even insignificant, should be noted. A lens should be used to get an accurate idea of the nature of edges, ends and floor of the wound.
Site	Record the anatomical position of the wound(s) with reference to some landmark, e.g., midline, bony structure, umbilicus.
Size	The dimensions of the wound(s) should be measured and never guessed, and amount of blood extravasated should be measured.
Shape	Describe the shape of the wound(s) (e.g., linear, curved, irregular, circular, oval or triangular) and also the beveling of the edges.
Surrounds	Note the condition of the surrounding or the nearby tissues (e.g., bruised, swollen).
Color	Observation of color is particularly relevant when describing bruises and abrasions.
Course	Comment on the apparent direction of the force applied (e.g., in abrasions and incised wounds) viz. horizontal, vertical or oblique with regard to anatomical position of the body.
Contents	Note the presence of any foreign material in the wound(s) (e.g., dirt, glass).
Age	Comment on any evidence of healing. Note that accurate ageing is impossible and great caution is required when commenting on this aspect.
Borders	The characteristics of the edges of the wound(s) may provide a clue as to the weapon used.
Depth	Give an indication of the depth of the wound(s); this may have to be an estimate.

Advice

- It is appropriate to mention the investigations, procedures and management of the patient.
- In all injuries, when fracture of a bone is suspected, an X-ray should be done for confirmation.

Samples and Specimens

- Samples and specimens collected should be properly identified, sealed and labeled.
- They should be kept in safe custody and handed over to the I.O. of the case.
- Specimens once collected, loss/destruction of evidence is a punishable offence.
- All evidence collected should be mentioned in MLR to establish the chain of custody in a court of law subsequently.

Opinion

What was the Type of Weapon Used?

- In many cases, examination of the wound and clothing give fairly definite information about the kind of weapon (hard blunt object/impact or sharp/blunt edged/pointed instrument or object).
- With stabs and incised wound, there is not much difficulty.

What was the Nature of the Injury?

- Opinion is given as to whether the injuries were simple or grievous in nature (as per **Sec. 116 BNS**).
- Against each injury, it should be noted whether it is simple or grievous.
- Injured person must be kept under observation, if nature of particular injury cannot be made out at the time of examination, e.g., head injury or abdominal injury.
- The initial or provisional report should be made available immediately.
- A subsequent report (supplementary report) should be given, once the investigation results become available — reflects the final conclusions drawn from the examination findings.
- Whether an injury is simple or grievous is decided on the basis of *status of injury at the time of infliction* and not after medical/surgical intervention.

What is the Time Passed Since Infliction of the Injury?

Opinion is based on the state of healing of the injuries as was recorded in the column of examination of the injuries.

What was the Manner of Infliction of Injury?

The history, clinical examination and findings on investigations and examination, all are considered together to opine whether the injuries sustained are consistent with alleged history [fall or road traffic accident (or any other accident) or assault].

MEDICO-LEGAL REPORT

(Instructions to Fill up MLR)

CR. No. ________________

Fill up all preliminary particulars

MLR No. ________________

Name ________________ S/D/W of ________________ Age ______ Gender ______

Residence ________________ Occupation ________________ Police Station ________________

Brought by ________________ Date and Time of Examination ________________

(If relative/friend—Name, address and signature)

Fill up date and time

Date and time of admission ________________

No. and date of police docket ________________

No. and name of constable ________________

History

History as narrated by the patient (if conscious) or relative (mention relation and take signature), date, time and place of incident

---

Articles handed over to the police

Mention the articles/clothing preserved

General condition (Vitals)

General condition, orientation to time, place and person, GCS, BP, Pulse, Temperature

Particulars of injuries

Type of injury + Dimension (use scale) + Location (in 2-D) + Characteristic features (including shape and orientation on skin surface—oblique/horizontal/vertical) + Healing changes + Any special remarks (foreign matter, etc.)

CONSENT

I am willing for my medico-legal examination.
I have not been examined medico-legally earlier.
I will show all my injuries on my person.
I have been explained that the result of the examination may go in my favor or against me.
All the information given is correct to the best of my knowledge.

Take consent from patient/relative (if patient is unconscious)

Signature/Thumb Impression of patient/guardian

Mention the advice given

Identification Marks

Write two ID marks

1. ________________

2. ________________

1. Nature of injuries

Keep under observations until sure

Opinion based on Sec. 116 BNS

(Simple/grievous)

2. Probable duration of injuries

6 or 12 or 24 hours or how many days

____

Kind of weapon used

- **Abrasion—Blunt/Pointed**
- **Lacerated wound/Contusion—Blunt**
- **Incised wound/Stab wound–Sharp**
- **Chop wound—Heavy and moderately sharp**
- **Firearm wound (Bullet—Rifle, Pellets–Shotgun)**

MEDICO-LEGAL REPORT

(Instructions to Fill up MLR)

CR. No. _____ XXXXX _____   MLR No. 12345/24

Name _____ Shamsher Singh _____ S/D/W of _____ Paramjeet Singh _____ Age 35 years Gender __ M __

Residence _____ H. No. 9871, Joshi Nagar, Haibowal, Ludhiana _____ Occupation _____ Car Dealer _____ Police Station _____ Haibowal

Brought by _____ Rataan Singh (Brother)—Same address as above _____ Date and Time of examination _____ 29/1/2024 at 9.05 pm

(If relative/friend—Name, address and signature)

Date and time of admission 29/1/2024 at 9.00 pm No. and date of police docket 29/1/2024 at 10.00 pm No. and name of constable Tejpreet Singh	**History:** Alleged H/o assault by group of people on 29/1/2024 at 8.30 pm when the patient was returning home from his showroom. There is no history of vomiting or loss of consciousness.

Articles handed over to the police

Shirt, vest and pant air dried, signed and packed in a cloth and put in a brown paper bag and sealed with 12 seals

General condition (Vitals): Patient is semi-conscious, barely able to talk, disoriented, GCS 12

BP—80/60 mm Hg, Pulse—110/min, RR—30/min

Pupils—B/L equal in size and reacting to light

Particulars of injuries:

1. Incised wound 6 × 0.5 cm × muscle deep present obliquely over the outer aspect of front of left upper arm, 15.5 cm below the tip of shoulder. Tailing is present at the lower end. Bleeding present. Shirt is having corresponding cut and is bloodstained.
2. Spindle shaped stab wound 3 × 0.5 cm (depth to be ascertained by surgeon) present vertically on the left side front of chest, 6 cm away from the midline and upper angle 9 cm below clavicle. Edges of the wound are clean cut and regular. Active bleeding present. Shirt and vest showing corresponding cut and is bloodstained. Advice chest X-ray, CT scan and surgery consult.
3. Lacerated wound 4.3 × 1.5 cm × bone deep present obliquely on the right side parietal region of the head, 7.5 cm above the pinna. Bleeding present. Advice CT scan head and neurosurgery consult.
4. Reddish abrasion 4 × 1.5 cm present over the front of right knee joint.

CONSENT

I am willing for my medico-legal examination.

I have not been examined medico-legally earlier.

I will show all my injuries on my person.

I have been explained that the result of the examination may go in my favor or against me.

All the information given is correct and to the best of my knowledge.

Signature/Thumb Impression of patient/guardian

Identification Marks	**1. Nature of injuries** 1 and 4 are simple (Simple/grievous) 2 is kept under observation and surgeon's opinion 3 is kept under observation for neurosurgeon's opinion 2. Probable duration of injuries Fresh (within 6 hours)	**Kind of weapon used** 1. Sharp 2. Pointed and sharp-edges both sides 3 and 4. Blunt (Dr Amit Kumar) PMC No. 12345 Signature of the Doctor Name, Designation and Seal
1. Linear glistening scar mark 3 × 0.5 cm obliquely present on the left side of face, 2 cm below the outer angle of eye. 2. Blackish mole 0.5 × 0.5 cm on the back left hand, 5 cm below the wrist joint.		

Date _29/1/2024_   **MLR No.** ___12345___   **CR No.** __XXXXX__

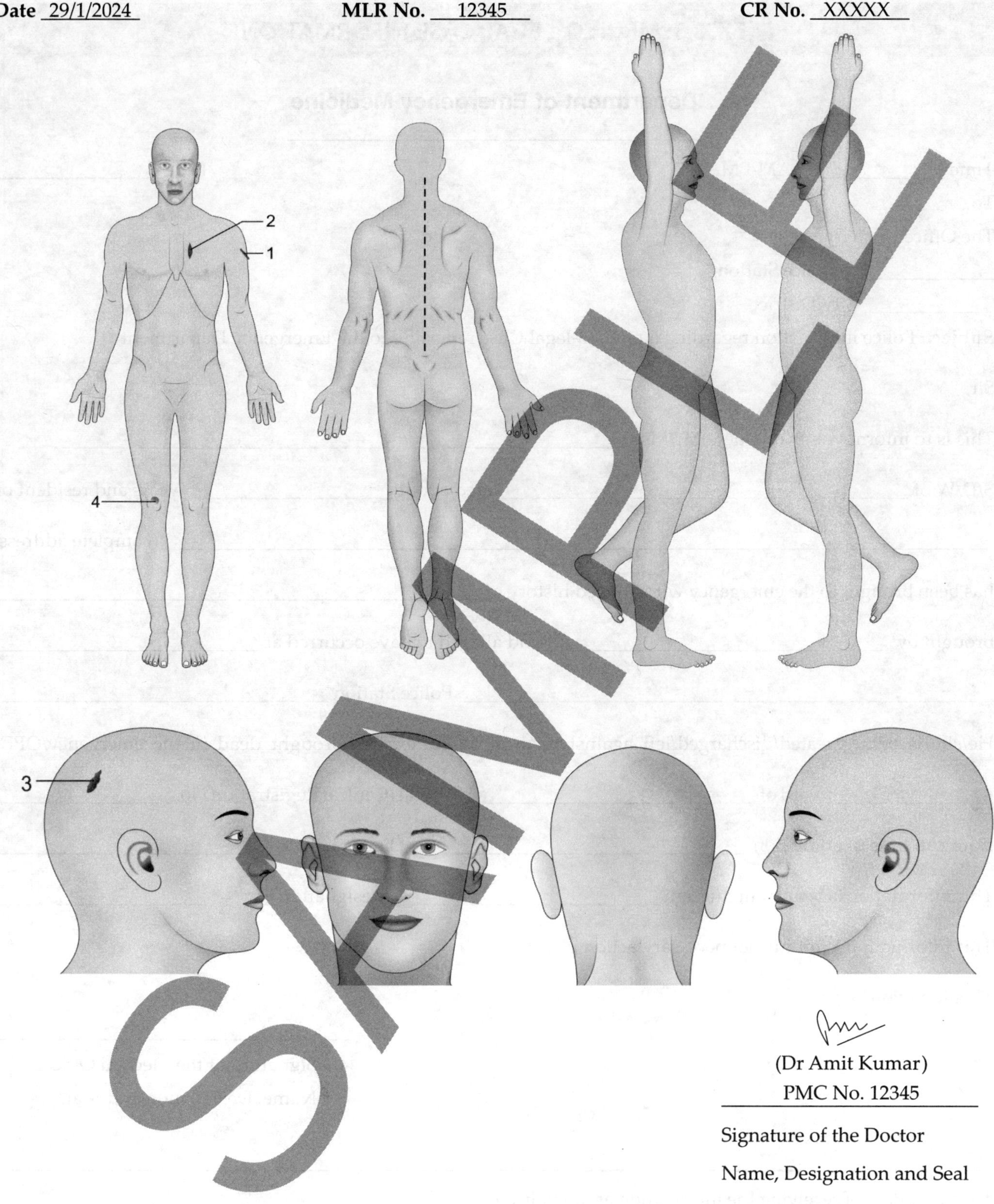

(Dr Amit Kumar)

_______PMC No. 12345_______

Signature of the Doctor

Name, Designation and Seal

EX. 3.3: MEDICO-LEGAL CASE INFORMATION

Department of Emergency Medicine

Time _______________ AM/PM   Date _______________

To

The Officer Incharge

_______________Police Station,

_______________ City/District

Subject: Police information regarding a medico-legal Case reporting to the Emergency Department

Sir,

This is to inform you that patient Mr/Ms ____

S/D/W of ____ aged about _____________________ years and resident of

____(complete address)

has been brought to the emergency with alleged history of____,

brought by ____ and alleged to have occurred at _______________________

____ Police Station _______________________________________.

He/she is being treated/discharged/left against medical advice/expired/brought dead in the emergency/OPD/

_______________ward of _________________________________ Hospital (Central Registration No. _______________).

Date and time of admission ____ Diagnosis _______________________________

This information is being sent through _____________________________ Designation _______________________________.

This information is for further necessary action please.

Thanking you.

____

Signature of the Medical Officer

Name, Designation and Seal

____

Time and date of receiving the information at the police post _______________________________

Signature of the Police Officer_______________________________

Name (in capital letters) _______________________________

Seal of the police post

EX. 3.4A: MEDICO-LEGAL REPORT I

FM 14.1: Examine and prepare medico-legal report of an injured person with different etiologies in a simulated/supervised environment.

Ankur Ranawat, a 38-year-old male while going to office on his motorcycle was hit by a car coming from opposite side at 10.00 AM. He was rushed to the emergency department of your hospital in unconscious state. Prepare a medico-legal report showing one simple and two grievous injuries on his person.

CR. No. _____________________ MLR No. _____________________

Name _____________________ S/D/W of _____________________ Age ______ Gender ______

Residence _____________________ Occupation ____________ Police Station _____________________

Brought by _____________________ Date and Time of examination _____________________
(If relative/friend—Name, address and signature)

Date and time of admission _____________________

No. and date of police docket _____________________

No. and name of constable _____________________

Articles handed over to the police

History

General condition (Vitals)

Particulars of injuries

CONSENT

I am willing for my medico-legal examination.
I have not been examined medico-legally earlier.
I will show all my injuries on my person.
I have been explained that the result of the examination may go in my favor or against me.
All the information given is correct to the best of my knowledge.

Signature/Thumb Impression of patient/guardian

Identification Marks	
1. _____________________	1. Nature of injuries _____________________ (Simple/grievous)
2. _____________________	2. Probable duration of injuries ____________

Kind of weapon used

Signature of the Doctor
Name, Designation and Seal

Date _________   **MLR No.** _________   **CR No.** _________

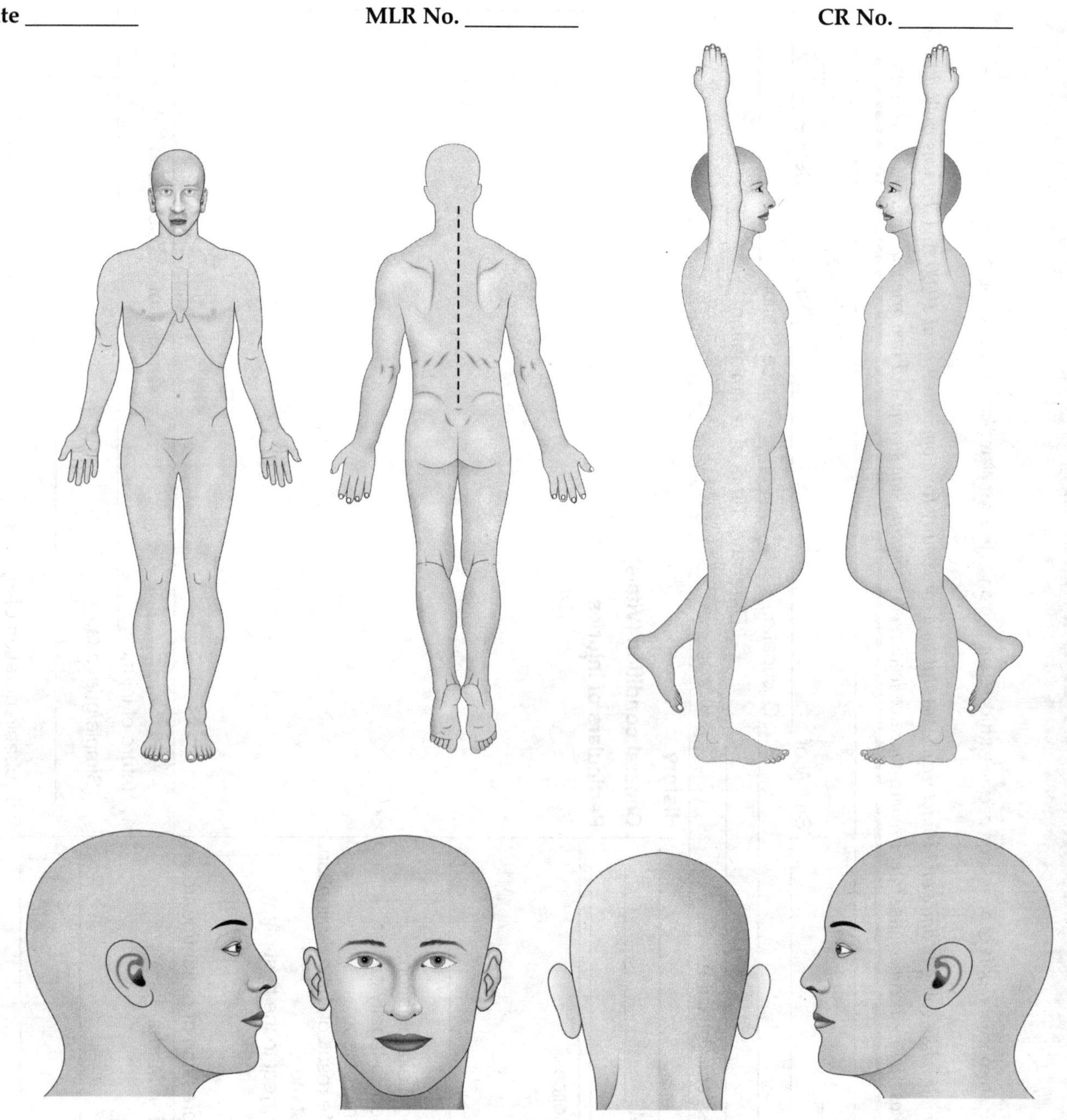

____

Signature of the Doctor

Name, Designation and Seal

EX. 3.4B: MEDICO-LEGAL REPORT II

FM 14.1: Examine and prepare medico-legal report of an injured person with different etiologies in a simulated/supervised environment.

Meera Devi, a 26-year-old female sustained second to third degree burns to her face and chest, entire left arm, anterior portion of her right arm and upper one-third of her abdomen when her in-laws and husband tried to burn her for dowry. She was rushed to the hospital by her neighbors. Remnants of burnt clothes were present on her body. Prepare a medico-legal report describing the burn injury.

CR. No. ______________________   MLR No. ____________________

Name __________________________________ S/D/W of ________________________________ Age ______ Gender ______

Residence ____ Occupation ____________ Police Station __________________

Brought by ______________________________________   Date and Time of examination ____________________

(If relative/friend—Name, address and signature)

Date and time of admission ____________________

No. and date of police docket ____________________

No. and name of constable ____________________

Articles handed over to the police

History

General condition (Vitals)

Particulars of injuries

CONSENT

I am willing for my medico-legal examination.
I have not been examined medico-legally earlier.
I will show all my injuries on my person.
I have been explained that the result of the examination may go in my favor or against me.
All the information given is correct to the best of my knowledge.

Signature/Thumb Impression of patient/guardian

Identification Marks

1. __________________________________

2. __________________________________

1. Nature of Injuries ____________________

   (Simple/grievous)

   ____

2. Probable duration of injuries ____________

   ____

Kind of weapon used

____

____

Signature of the Doctor
Name, Designation and Seal

Date __________ **MLR No.** __________ **CR No.** __________

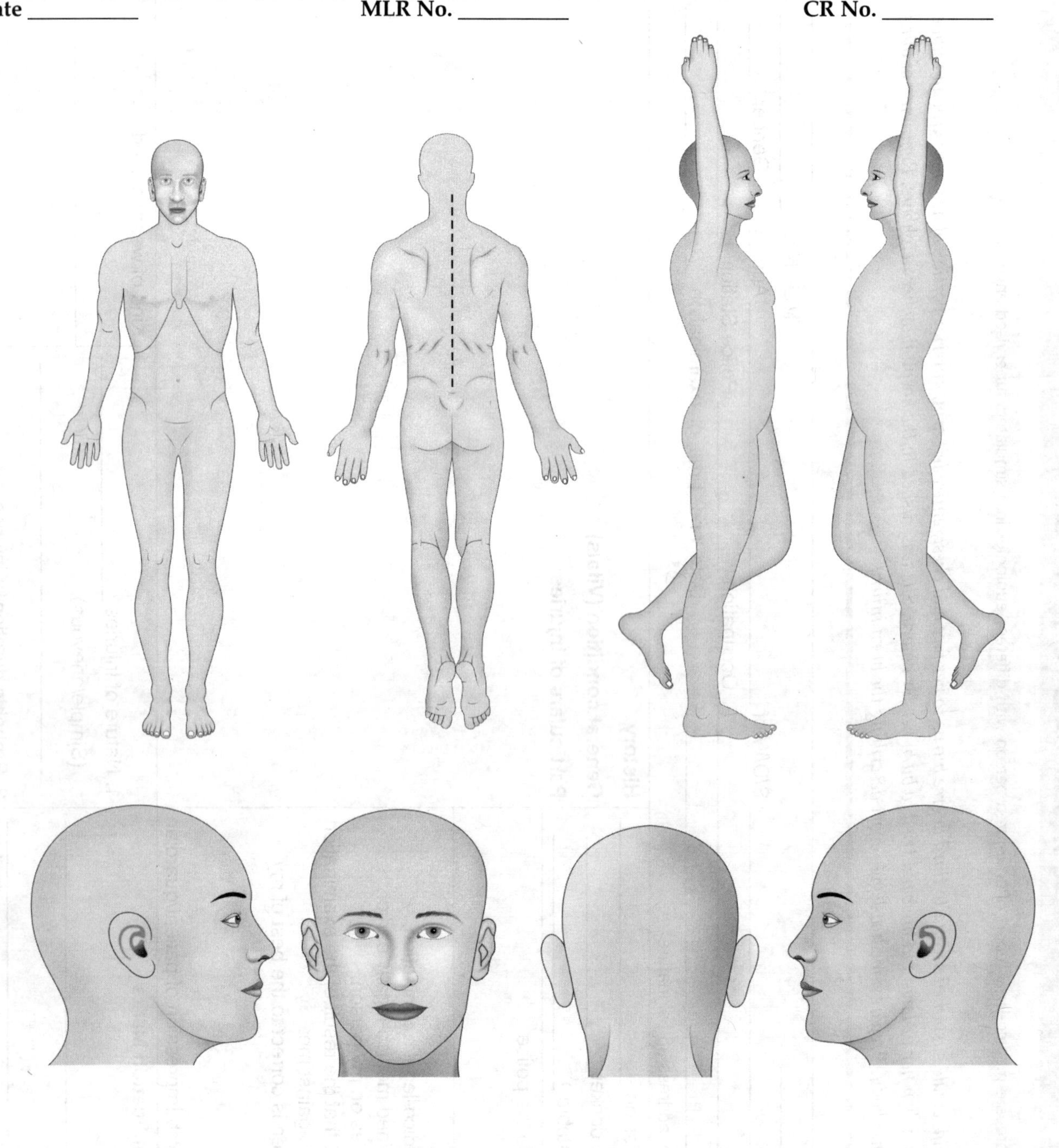

Signature of the Doctor

Name, Designation and Seal

EX. 3.4C: MEDICO-LEGAL REPORT III

FM 14.1: Examine and prepare medico-legal report of an injured person with different etiologies in a simulated/supervised environment.

A 36-year-old married female was allegedly assaulted by an unknown person with a knife when he tried to snatch her purse. She was brought to the casualty department with an elliptical stab wound on the left side of her chest and an incised wound on the left arm. Her vitals were B.P. 102/70 mm Hg, pulse: 92/min, respiratory rate: 22/min, and GCS: 15/15. She was wearing salwar kameez, bra and panty. Prepare a medico-legal report for the same.

CR. No. _________________________   MLR No. _________________________

Name _________________________ S/D/W of _________________________ Age ______ Gender ______

Residence _________________________ Occupation _____________ Police Station _________________

Brought by _________________________   Date and Time of examination _________________

(If relative/friend—Name, address and signature)

Date and time of admission _________________	**History**
No. and date of police docket _________________	**General condition (Vitals)**
No. and name of constable _________________	**Particulars of injuries**
Articles handed over to the police	

CONSENT

I am willing for my medico-legal examination.
I have not been examined medico-legally earlier.
I will show all my injuries on my person.
I have been explained that the result of the examination may go in my favor or against me.
All the information given is correct to the best of my knowledge.

Signature/Thumb Impression of patient/guardian

Identification Marks		
1. _________________________	1. Nature of injuries _________________ (Simple/grievous) _________________	**Kind of weapon used** _________________
2. _________________________	2. Probable duration of injuries _________ _________________	_________________ Signature of the Doctor Name, Designation and Seal

Date ______________ **MLR No.** ______________ **CR No.** ______________

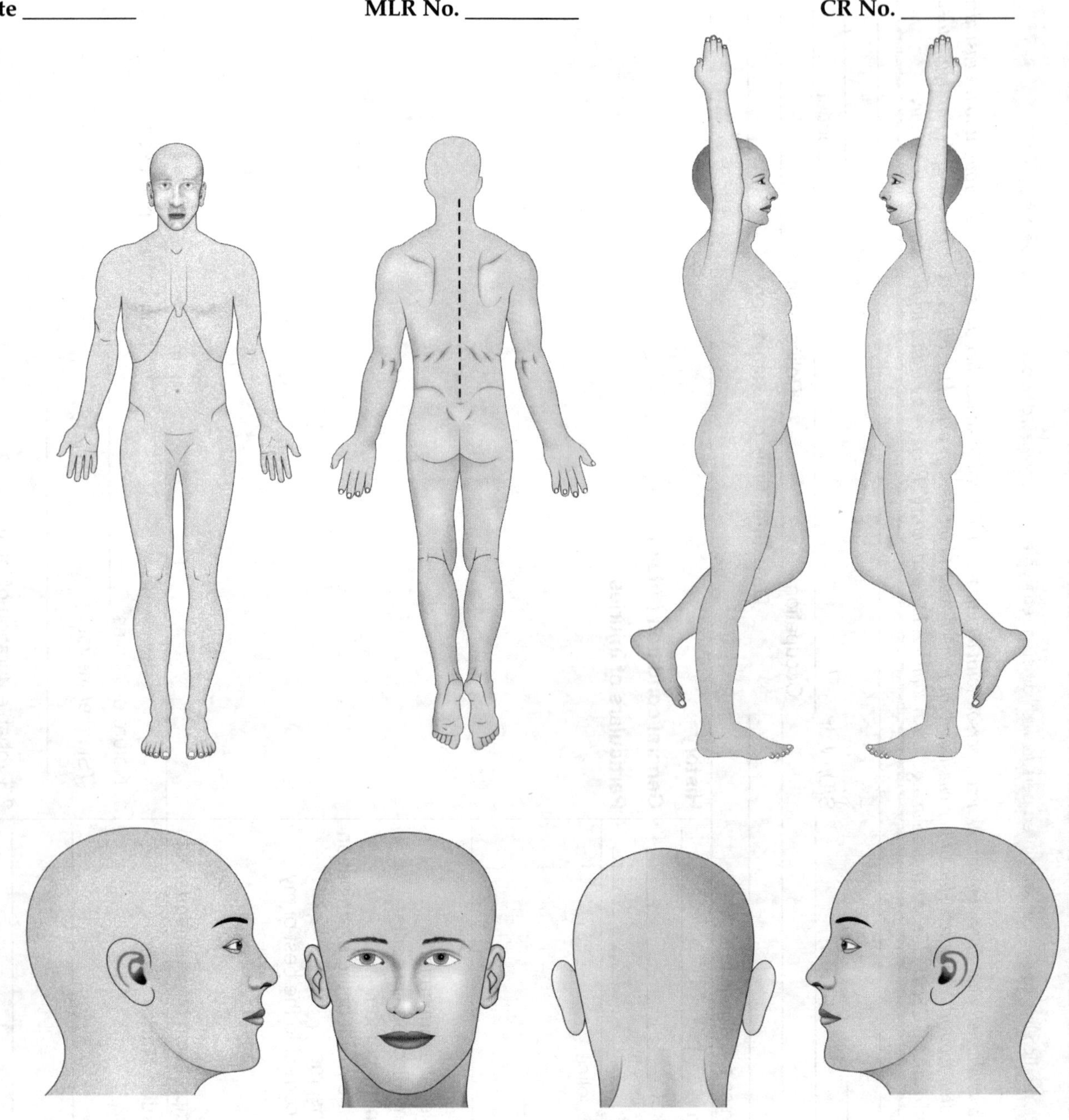

Signature of the Doctor

Name, Designation and Seal

EX. 3.4D: MEDICO-LEGAL REPORT IV

FM 14.1: Examine and prepare medico-legal report of an injured person with different etiologies in a simulated/supervised environment.

Dr Mani Venkataraman, a 56-year-old doctor suffered multiple gunshot injuries from an assault by an unknown person at about 5.30–5.45 AM while on his morning walk, when the person approached him and started shooting indiscriminately from a close range. He was immediately rushed to the hospital. There was one entry wound on right lateral chest wall in mid-axillary line and two entry and two exit bullet wounds on the right upper arm. He was wearing a track suit, vest and briefs at the time of incident. Prepare a medico-legal report for the same.

CR. No. _______________   MLR No. _______________

Name _______________ S/D/W of _______________ Age ______ Gender ______

Residence _______________ Occupation _______________ Police Station _______________

Brought by _______________   Date and Time of examination _______________

(If relative/friend—Name, address and signature)

Date and time of admission _______________	**History**
No. and date of police docket _______________	**General condition (Vitals)**
No. and name of constable _______________	**Particulars of injuries**
Articles handed over to the police	
CONSENT I am willing for my medico-legal examination. I have not been examined medico-legally earlier. I will show all my injuries on my person. I have been explained that the result of the examination may go in my favor or against me. All the information given is correct to the best of my knowledge. Signature/Thumb Impression of patient/guardian	

Identification Marks	1. Nature of Injuries _______________ (Simple/grievous) _______________ 2. Probable duration of injuries _______________	Kind of weapon used _______________ Signature of the Doctor Name, Designation and Seal
1. _______________ 2. _______________		

Date _________   MLR No. _________   CR No. _________

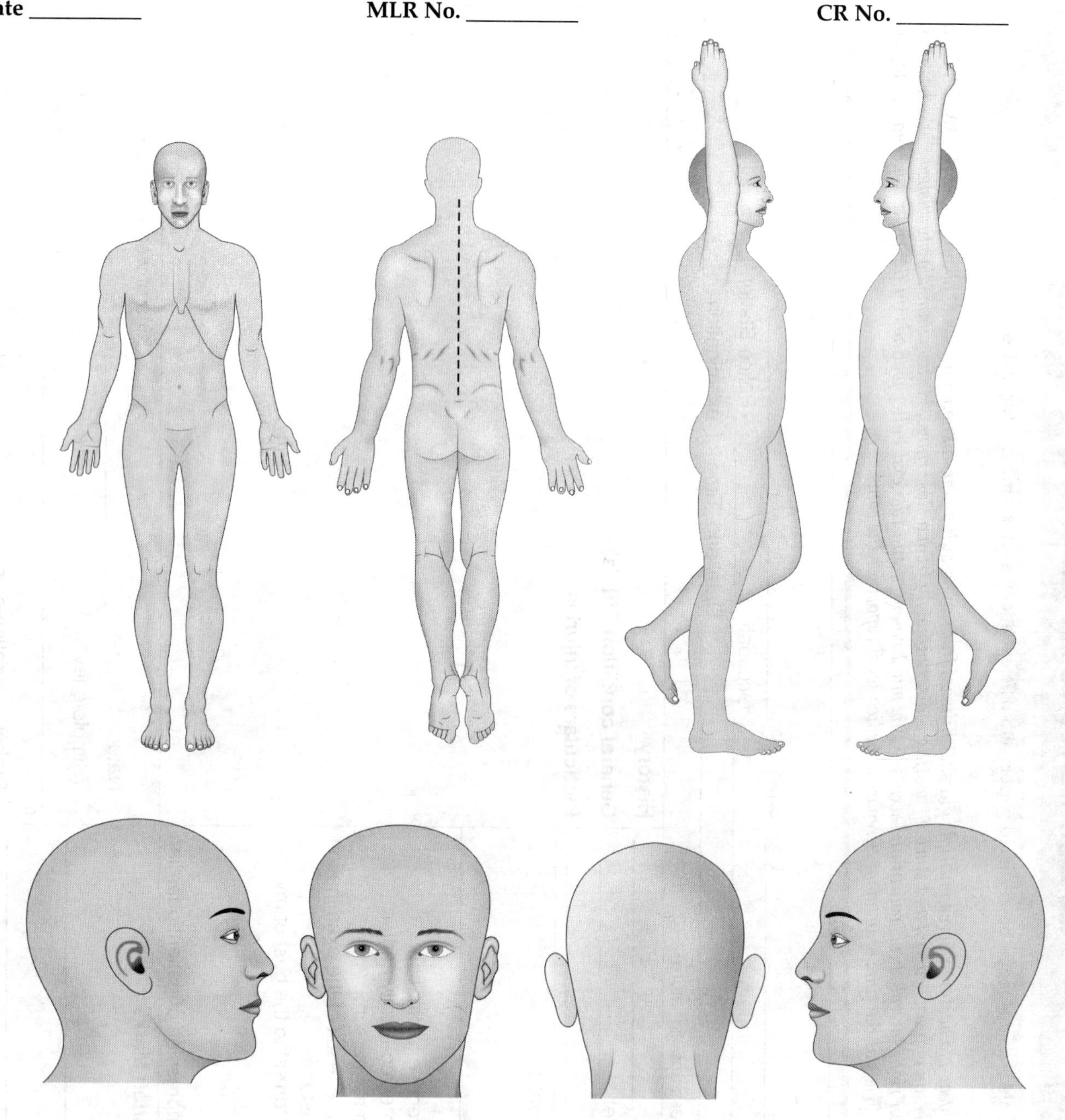

Signature of the Doctor

Name, Designation and Seal

EX. 3.4E: MEDICO-LEGAL REPORT V

CR. No. ___________________

MLR No. ___________________

Name _________________________________ S/D/W of _________________________________ Age ______ Gender ______

Residence _________________________________ Occupation ___________ Police Station ___________________

Brought by _________________________________

Date and Time of Examination ___________________

(If relative/friend—Name, address and signature)

Date and time of admission ___________________

No. and date of police docket ___________________

No. and name of constable ___________________

Articles handed over to the police

History

General condition (Vitals)

Particulars of injuries

CONSENT

I am willing for my medico-legal examination.
I have not been examined medico-legally earlier.
I will show all my injuries on my person.
I have been explained that the result of the examination may go in my favor or against me.
All the information given is correct to the best of my knowledge.

Signature/Thumb Impression of patient/guardian

Identification Marks

1. ___________________

2. ___________________

1. Nature of injuries ___________________
   (Simple/grievous)

   ____

2. Probable duration of injuries ___________

   ____

Kind of weapon used

____

____

Signature of the Doctor
Name, Designation and Seal

Date __________   **MLR No.** __________   **CR No.** __________

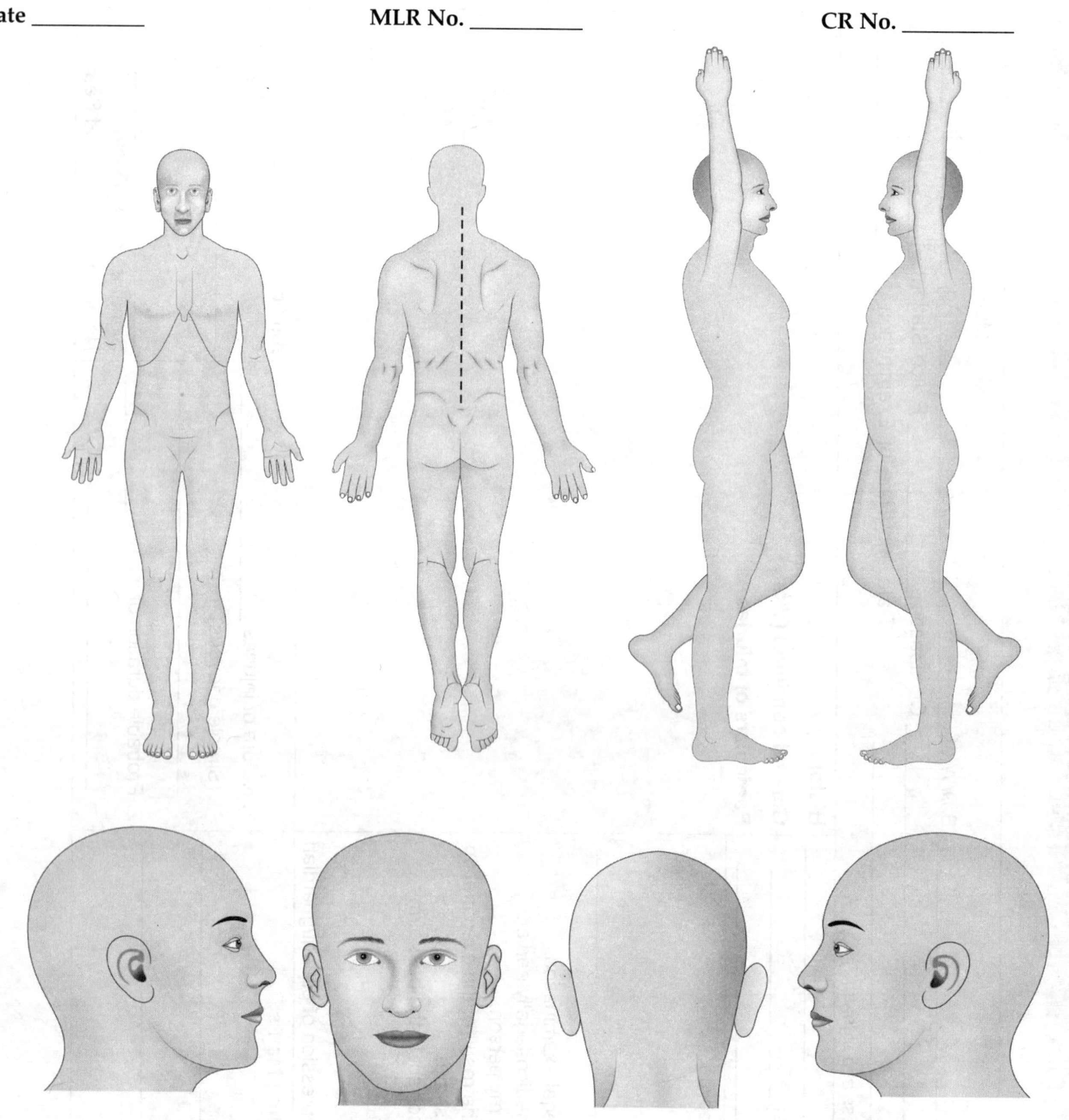

Signature of the Doctor

Name, Designation and Seal

EX. 3.5: REQUISITION FORM FOR INVESTIGATIONS

Department of Forensic Medicine and Toxicology

____

To   Date ______________

The Professor/Medical Officer I/C

Department of Radiology/Pathology/Biochemistry

____

Subject: X ray/CT/USG/MRI scan/Laboratory investigation required

Dear Sir/Madam,

Ref.: MLC No. __________________ CR No. __________________ Dated __________________

I request that radiograph/CT/USG/MRI/_________________________________ (investigations) of the subject

Mr/Ms _______________________ aged _________ years, resident of _________________________________

may be taken/carried out as indicated below:

1.   ____

2.   ____

3.   ____

Brief history: ____

____

____

The subject bears the following identification marks:

1.   ____

2.   ____

I request you that the report and opinion may be sent to the undersigned at the earliest.

Thanking you

With regards,

____

Signature of the Doctor

Name, Designation and Seal

Place ______________

Date ______________

EX. 3.6: SUPPLEMENTARY REPORT

Department of Forensic Medicine and Toxicology

To   Date ________________

The Investigating Officer,

________________________ Police Station,

________________District/City/Town

Subject: Supplementary report in case of Mr/Ms ____

S/D/W of ______________________________ vide MLR No. ______________________ dated ________________

Sir,

Keeping in view the ______________________ report nos. ______________________, I am of the opinion that

injury nos. ______________________ are simple in nature, and injury nos. ______________ are grievous in nature.

With regards,

____

Signature of the doctor

Name, Designation and Seal

Enclosed: *(Tick '√')*

☐ ____________ X-rays along with report in original duly initialed by me
☐ ____________ CT along with report in original duly initialed by me
☐ Surgeon's report in original duly initialed by me
☐ Pathology report in original duly initialed by me

____

Received supplementary report along with ________________ X-rays and/or ________________ report(s).

Name ______________________________ P.C. No. ______________________ P.S. ______________

____

Signature and Date

EX. 3.7: EXAMINATION REPORT OF A WEAPON

FM 14.10: Prepare a report of the weapon brought by police and give opinion regarding injuries present on the person as described in injury report/PM report so as to connect weapon with the injuries.
(Correlate with injury report No. 3 to connect the weapon with the injuries)

Department of Forensic Medicine and Toxicology

____

To

The Investigation Officer,

____________________ (Police Station)

____________________ (Place)

Subject: Examination of the weapon provided (Reference letter No. ____

dated ______________________________)

Sir/Madam

In reference to the above letter, I am sending you the report about the weapon sent in a parcel with _____________

seals in connection with the injuries sustained by Mr/Ms _________________ S/D/W of _____________________

aged about _____________ years (vide MLR No. _________________ dated __________________________).

Description of the Weapon
(The weapon should preferably be examined after fingerprint and serological examination)

Name of weapon ____________________   Type of weapon ___________________

Shape (refer to the diagram) ______________________

Weapon (intact/broken) ______________________

Weight ____________________

(in case of heavy blunt object)

Length _____________   Width/Circumference ___________________

Thickness/diameter ____________________

Edges (margins)/surface ____________________

Tip/end ____________________

Handle ____________________

Joint _______________ Type _____________

Hilt ____________________

Trace evidence (hair/fibers/cloth/stains/rust), if any ____________________________________

Injuries possible ____

Identification marks, if any, on the weapon ____________________________________

Labeled Diagram

(Put signature and date with indelible ink on the weapon)

Opinion (*may be framed from any of the given sentences*)

- After examination of the weapon, I am of the opinion that injury No(s) _______, _______, _______, _______, is/are possible with the given weapon.
- After examination of the weapon, I am of the opinion that injury No(s) _______, _______, _______, _______, is/are not possible with the given weapon.
- After examination of the weapon, I am of the opinion that none/all of the injuries mentioned are possible/are not possible with the given weapon.

____

Place _______________   Signature of the Doctor

Date _______________   Name, Designation and Seal

____

Received report along with the weapon packed and sealed with ___________ seals.

Name ____ P.C. No. _________________________ P.S. _____________________

____

Signature and Date

EX. 3.8: MEDICO-LEGAL REPORT IN CASE OF POISONING

FM 14.2: Demonstrate the correct technique of clinical examination in a suspected case of poisoning and prepare medico-legal report in a simulated/supervised environment.

Manju Deshwal, a 21-year-old female, was brought to the emergency in unconscious state, with alleged history of ingestion of 20–25 tablets of benzodiazepines tablets 3 hours back. Off late, she was under stress, and tried to commit suicide because of breach of promise to marry by her partner. On examination, her GCS was 3, mild cyanosis and pallor was present. Pulse: 100/min feeble, B.P. 82/mm Hg systolic, respiratory rate 28/min regular, Temperature - 36.4 °C. CNS examination showed deep coma, bilateral constricted pupils, which reacted minimally to light; diminished tendon reflexes and plantar reflexes were not elicitable bilaterally with retention of urine. There was no response to painful stimuli. Prepare a medico-legal report for the same.

Department of Forensic Medicine and Toxicology

MLR No. ________________   Date and time of examination ____________

Name ____ S/D/W of ________________________

Age __________ years   Gender ____________________

Address ____

Brought by ________________________________ Relation ____________________

Consent	Marks of Identification
I am willing for my medico-legal examination. I have not been examined medico-legally earlier. I have been explained that the result of the examination may go in my favor or against. All the information given is correct to best of my knowledge. Signature/Thumb Impression of the person/guardian	1. ________________________________ ________________________________ 2. ________________________________ ________________________________

Brief history the case: (Name of the person giving history ________________________________)

(including symptoms, quantity, route, manner of exposure, date and time of onset)

____

____

____

____

Findings of Medical Examination

Clothings ____

Pulse _________/min   B.P. _________ mm Hg   Respiratory rate _________/min

Temperature _____ °C   GCS ____________

Consciousness	☐ Fully conscious	☐ Drowsy	☐ Unconscious
Orientation (time, place, person)	☐ Well oriented	☐ Disoriented	
Memory (recent/remote)	☐ Intact	☐ Impaired	
Mental status	☐ Normal ☐ Delirious	☐ Depressed ☐ Seizures (generalized/partial)	☐ Agitated
Condition of skin	☐ Flushed ☐ Rash ☐ Discolored __________	☐ Pale ☐ Blisters	☐ Dry ☐ Perspiration
Needle marks/bite marks	☐ Absent	☐ Present (describe) __________	
Eyes (conjunctivae)	☐ Normal	☐ Congested	
Pupils	☐ Normal	☐ Dilated	☐ Constricted
Mouth/lips/tongue	☐ Normal ☐ Bitten	☐ Moist ☐ Discolored	☐ Dry
Smell from expired breath	☐ Absent ☐ Present (garlicky/kerosene-like/fruity/rotten eggs/phenolic/burnt rope/ bitter almonds/__________)		
Vomitus (note color, odor, amount)			
Urine/stool (note color, consistency)			

(Tick '✓')

Systemic Examination

Central nervous system ____

Reflexes ____

Chest ____

Abdomen ____

Material Preserved: Blood/urine/vomitus/stool/clothes/suicidal note (if found)

(Tick '√')

Advice ____

Opinion is reserved till receipt of chemical examiner's report with regards to kind of poison.

Place ______________

Date ______________

____

Signature of the Doctor

Name, Designation and Seal

EX. 3.9: DISPATCH OF SAMPLES

FM 14.3: Assist and demonstrate the proper technique in collecting, preserving and dispatch of the exhibits in a suspected case of poisoning, along with clinical examination.

Madhavan, a 45-year-old male presented with an alleged history of ingestion of a few drops of dichlorvos which was followed by multiple episodes of vomiting and breathing difficulty. There was no history of seizure, loss of consciousness or chest pain. On examination, he was conscious, but restless, no focal deficit, no nuchal rigidity, with bilateral pinpoint pupils. His vitals were BP 150/80 mm Hg, pulse 60/minute, tachypnea with respiratory rate 30/minute, random blood sugar 200 mg%, with excessive oral secretions, and bilateral crepitation. Identify the samples to be taken and preserved for investigation and diagnosis.

Department of Forensic Medicine and Toxicology

FMT No._____________	**TOXICOLOGICAL REQUEST**	Use capital letters to fill the form **Ante-mortem □ Post-mortem □**

MLR No. ___________________________ Date and time of sampling _________________________

Name _______________________________S/ D/ W of _______________________________

Age __________ years   Gender _____________________ Occupation___________________

Address ____

Brought by _______________________________ Relation ___________________________

Consent	**Marks of Identification**
I am willing for my medico-legal examination. I have not been examined earlier. I have been explained that the result of the examination may go in my favor or against. Signature/ Thumb Impression of the person/ guardian	1. _________________________ _________________________ 2. _________________________ _________________________

Suspected Etiology

Driving accident □   Driver □   Pedestrian □   Passenger □

Homicide □   Suicide □   Home/leisure accident □

Occupational accident □   Unknown □

Other ____

Cause of death (if known): ____

Toxicological Request Reason

Intoxication suspicion: Yes □ No □ If no, give brief details:________________________

Apparent natural death □   Death with traumatic lesions □ Drug abuse □ Rape and homicide

Other:____

Requested Analysis

*Medicines ☐ *Pesticides ☐ *Drugs of abuse ☐ Ethyl alcohol ☐ Carbon monoxide ☐

*Other____

*Mention whenever it is possible, the xenobiotic/poison suspected.

Was any toxicological analyses performed before on either ante- or post-mortem samples?

Yes ☐ No ☐

If yes, give details of the results:____

Past or Recent Medical History

Details of any recent history of illness/disease_______________________________________

Any prescribed drugs____

Are the specimens likely to be infected with HIV, tuberculosis, hepatitis or any other serious disease?

Yes ☐ No ☐ If yes, give details:____

Current History of Poisoning/Intoxication

Time/Date of: Intoxication___________________, onset of symptoms/signs___________________, hospital
admission___________________, when last seen alive:_______________, when body found:___________

Circumstances in which intoxication occurred: _____________________________________

____

____

Relevant symptoms: Diarrhea ☐ Vomiting ☐ Thirst ☐ Pain ☐ Blindness ☐ Constipation ☐ Tremors ☐

Cyanosis ☐ Jaundice ☐ Loss of weight ☐ Shivering ☐ Sweating ☐ Convulsions ☐ Miosis ☐ Mydriasis ☐

Delirium ☐ Coma ☐

Affected organs, which:_____________________ Others: Give details:_____________________

____

Was any medical treatment or first aid given? Yes ☐ No ☐

If yes, please provide details on the drug/medication given:_____________________________

____

Clinical features immediately before death (if applicable):_____________________________

Time/Date of death (if applicable):____

Where was the victim found (e.g., at work, in bed, outdoor):____________________________

Did he/she seem normal when last seen alive: Yes ☐ No ☐ If not, give brief details:___________

Samples for Analysis

Sample		Number	Time*	Quantity
Blood	Peripheral Cardiac Other			
Urine				
Bile				
Vitreous humor				
Organs	Stomach and intestines Liver Kidney Brain Lung Others			
Gastric content (e.g., vomit and gastric lavage or aspirate)				
Others				

Time(s)/Date(s) of collection are particularly important for any samples taken prior to death, which are now being submitted for analysis.

Advice____

Opinion is reserved till receipt of chemical examiner's report with regards to kind of poison.

Place _____________

Date _____________

____
Signature of the Doctor

Name, Designation and Seal

A copy of any preliminary pathology report should be provided, if available. Report sent: Yes ☐ No ☐

Samples preserved for CFSL to be sealed and handed over to the police constable after taking a receipt.

EX. 3.10: EXAMINATION OF A CASE OF DRUNKENNESS

FM 14.15: To examine and prepare medico-legal report of a drunk person in a simulated/supervised environment.

Truck driver Sarma Chaudhary, a 48-year-old male was allegedly involved in a road side accident wherein he crushed two laborers under the wheels of his truck who were sleeping on the pavement. Upon arrival at the accident scene at 2 AM, the police officer found him shouting meaninglessly and detected an alcoholic odor from his breath, bloodshot eyes and slurred speech. An inspection of his truck revealed 2 empty whiskey bottles. He stated that he had consumed '2 or 3 pegs' 2 to 3 hours prior to the accident. He was arrested for driving under the influence of alcohol (Sec. 185 Motor Vehicle Act) and Sec. 304A IPC, and brought for medico-legal examination. Prepare a report for the same.

Department of Forensic Medicine and Toxicology

MLR No. ________________   C.R. No. ________________

Patient Details

Name ________________________________   S/ D/ W of ________________________

Address ____

Gender ________________   Age (as reported) __________ years

Educational status ____________________   Occupation ____________________

Examination Details

Date and time of examination ____________________ Time of completion ____________________

Requisition from ____________________ Vide letter no. __________ Dated ____________________

Brought by (Name and signature) ____________________ P.C. No.__________ P.S.__________

Accompanied by (name and relation) ____________________________________

Informed Consent

I, ____________________________ S/D/W of ____________________________ hereby agree for a complete physical examination, recording of findings, collection of specimens as necessary for laboratory analysis and any other investigations as recommended by the examining doctor and release of a report to the police officials/ court of law concerned. This procedure has been fully explained to me. Further, I have been explained that the result may go against me. This information may be used for teaching and research purposes provided no identifying data is released.

The above has been explained to me in ____________________language and I have fully understood the same and I am signing this consent by my own free will.

____

Signature and name of the witness

Address ________________

____

Signature/Thumb impression of patient/guardian

Marks of Identification

1. ____

2. ____

Brief history of the case ____

____

Narrated by ____

Medical History

Current medical problems ____

Past medical history ____

Hearing problems ____

Visual problems ____Use of spectacles/Contact lens: Yes/No

Balance problems ____

Diabetes: Yes/No   If taking insulin, when and how much taken ________________________

Epilepsy: Yes/No   Renal impairment: Yes/No   Hepatic impairment: Yes/No

Prescribed medication ____

Specific History of Alcohol Intake

Quantity of alcohol consumed in last 24 hours ______________   Type of liquor ____________________

First drink at ____________ AM/PM   Last drink at ____________ AM/PM

Last meal ____________ AM/PM   Type of meal ____________________

Weekly alcohol intake ____

Drug/addiction ____

Past psychiatric history ____

Past self-harm attempts ____

Previous trauma (particularly to head and extremities) ________________________

Social history ____

Family history ____

General Physical Examination

Built: Well/Average/Poor Height _______ cm Weight _______ kg

Pulse _______/min BP _______ mm Hg Respiratory rate _____/min

Areas of the body examined (*note injuries on separate body diagrams*) _______________________________

____

Clothing	☐ Decent	☐ Soiled	☐ Torn	☐ Disordered
Demeanor/behavior	☐ Sober ☐ Aggressive	☐ Abusive ☐ Boastful	☐ Talkative ☐ Calm	
Face	☐ Normal	☐ Flushed	☐ Pale	

Eyes
Conjunctiva
Pupils
    Reaction to light
Visual acuity
Nystagmus
    Horizontal gaze
    Vertical gaze
Convergence
	☐ Normal
	☐ Normal
	☐ Normal
	☐ Normal
	
	☐ Coarse
	☐ Yes
	☐ Yes
		☐ Congested
		☐ Dilated
		☐ Delayed
		☐ Abnormal
		
		☐ Fine
		☐ No
		☐ No
			☐ Contracted
			☐ Sluggishly reacting ☐ Non-reacting
			
			☐ Continuous
				
				☐ Absent

Ear (discharge)	☐ Yes	☐ No		
Mouth (signs of vomiting, salivation)	☐ Yes	☐ No		
Smell of alcohol	☐ Strong	☐ Moderate	☐ Faint	☐ None
Tongue	☐ Dry	☐ Moist	☐ Clean	☐ Furred
Speech	☐ Normal ☐ Overprecise	☐ Incoherent ☐ Thick and slurred	☐ Stuttering	
Gait	☐ Normal	☐ Broad-gauge	☐ Stumbling	☐ Self-control
Reflexes	☐ Normal	☐ Exaggerated	☐ Depressed (sluggish)	

Mental state
Self-control
Memory
Orientation
    Time
    Place
Reaction time
	☐ Normal
	☐ Clear
	
	☐ Good
	☐ Good
	☐ Normal
		☐ Impaired
		☐ Vague
		
		☐ Moderate
		☐ Moderate
		☐ Delayed
			
			☐ Confused
			
			☐ Bad
			☐ Bad
			☐ Increased
				
				☐ Indefinite
				☐ Indefinite

Drug abuse	☐ Needle marks ☐ Shivering ☐ Rhinorrhea ☐ Gooseflesh	☐ Yawning ☐ Lachrymation		

(*Tick '✓'*)

Specimen of handwriting ____

Impairment Tests *(to determine incoordination)*

1. Romberg's Test				
Able to stand still during instructions	☐ Yes	☐ No		
Body swaying	☐ Marked	☐ Moderate	☐ Minimal	☐ Absent
Able to complete the test	☐ Yes	☐ No		
2. Walk and Turn Test				
Able to stand still during instructions	☐ Yes	☐ No		
Start too soon	☐ Yes	☐ No		
Stops walking	☐ Yes	☐ No		
Misses heel/toe	☐ Yes	☐ No		
Gait on turning	☐ Normal	☐ Unsteady	☐ Stumbling	
Steps off line	☐ Yes	☐ No		
3. One Leg Stand Test				
Body swaying	☐ Marked	☐ Moderate	☐ Minimal	☐ Absent
Puts foot down	☐ Yes	☐ No		
Hops	☐ Yes	☐ No		
4. Finger and Nose Test				
Body swaying	☐ Marked	☐ Moderate	☐ Minimal	☐ Absent
Correct hand use	☐ Yes	☐ No		
Hand movements (incoordination)	☐ Marked	☐ Moderate	☐ Minimal	☐ Absent

(Tick '✓')

Systemic Examination

Cardiovascular system (heart sounds) ____

Respiratory system (PN, breath sounds, added sounds) ____

GIT Examination (Soft/Tender/Liver, Spleen, Kidneys/Bowel sounds) ____

____

Blood alcohol level (using breathalyzer or biochemical examination) _________________ mg%.

Sample preserved: Blood (in sodium fluoride and potassium oxalate) and urine (sodium fluoride) for FSL examination.

Opinion

Based on clinical and chemical examination, I am of the opinion that the above person has:

- ☐ Consumed alcohol and is under the influence of it.
- ☐ Consumed alcohol but is not under its influence.
- ☐ Not consumed alcohol.

(Tick '✓')

Place _____________

Date _____________

____

Signature of the Doctor

Name, Designation and Seal

Received MLR No. ____ along with a sealed glass vial, sample seal and an envelope addressed to chemical examiner.

Name _________________________________ P.C. No. _____________________ P.S. _______________________

____

Signature and Date

UNIT 4

Sexual Offences

EXAMINATION OF SURVIVOR

Survivor: The term 'survivor' is preferably used instead of 'victim' since it recognizes that the person is capable of taking decisions despite being victimized, humiliated and traumatized due to the assault.

It must be understood that forensic medical examination of the victim is a 'medico-legal emergency' as per the Supreme Court guidelines. Hence, such cases must be examined without delay. No such case should be refused for examination for the reasons of nonavailability of lady medical officer, because as per Sec. 184 Bharatiya Nagarik Suraksha Sanhita (BNSS), any registered medical practitioner (RMP) can examine survivor in presence of other woman with the consent of the patient or guardian.

Medical Examination of the Victim of Rape (Sec. 184 BNSS)

1. Where, during the stage when an offence of committing rape or attempt to commit rape is under investigation, it is proposed to get the woman with whom rape is alleged or attempted to have been committed or attempted, examined by a medical expert, such examination shall be conducted by a RMP employed in a hospital run by the Government or a local authority and in the absence of a such a practitioner, by any other RMP, with the consent of such woman or of a person competent to give such consent on her behalf and such woman shall be sent to such RMP within 24 hours from the time of receiving the information relating to the commission of such offence.
2. The RMP, to whom such woman is sent shall, without delay, examine her and prepare a report of his/her examination giving the following particulars, namely:
   a. The name and address of the woman and of the person by whom she was brought;
   b. The age of the woman;
   c. The description of material taken from the person of the woman for DNA profiling;
   d. Marks of injury, if any, on the person of the woman;
   e. General mental condition of the woman; and
   f. Other material particulars in reasonable detail.
3. The report shall state precisely the reasons for each conclusion arrived at.
4. The report shall specifically record that the consent of the woman or of the person competent to give such consent on her behalf to such examination had been obtained.
5. The exact time of commencement and completion of the examination shall also be noted in the report.
6. The RMP shall, without delay forward the report to the investigation officer who shall forward it to the Magistrate.
7. Nothing in this section shall be construed as rendering lawful any examination without the consent of the woman or of any person competent to give such consent on her behalf.

Explanation: For the purposes of this section, 'examination' and 'registered medical practitioner' shall have the same meanings as in Sec. 51 BNSS.

'Two-finger test': The Supreme Court has described this test to determine the 'laxity' of vagina as *'unscientific, inhuman and degrading'*. It cannot be used against a woman, and that a rape survivor's 'habituation to sexual intercourse' is immaterial. The test is often used by defendant's lawyer to label victims as 'loose women', and identified as being 'habituated to sex'.

The samples must be collected as per time elapsed between assault and examination, history and physical findings. This will avoid unnecessary sample collection.

The *provisional opinion* must, in brief, mention relevant aspects of the history of sexual violence, clinical findings and samples which are sent for analysis to Forensic science laboratory (FSL). The report should contain negative as well as positive findings. An inference must be drawn in the opinion, correlating the history and clinical findings **(Table 4.1)**. Absence of body/genital injuries on victim of sexual assault does not rule out commission of the offence.

The *final opinion* of whether sexual intercourse has taken place or not is based on a consideration of **(Table 4.1)**:

a. Signs of struggle.
b. Presence of blood and/or seminal stains on clothes and body.
c. Presence of seminal matter in the vagina.
d. Transmission of venereal disease.
e. Forensic science laboratory reports.

EXAMINATION OF ACCUSED

Examination of Accused by Medical Practitioner at the Request of Police Officer

1. When a person is arrested on a charge of committing an offence of such a nature and alleged to have been committed under such circumstances that there are reasonable grounds for believing that an examination of his person will afford evidence as to the commission of an offence, it shall be lawful for a RMP, acting at the request of a police officer, and for any person acting in good faith in his aid and under his direction, to make such an examination of the person arrested as is reasonable necessary in order to ascertain the facts which may afford such evidence, and to use such force as is reasonably necessary for that purpose **[Sec. 51(1) BNSS]**.
2. Whenever the person of a female is to be examined under this section, the examination shall be made only by, or under the supervision of, a female RMP **[Sec. 51(2) BNSS]**.

Examination of Accused of Rape by Medical Practitioner (Sec. 52 BNSS)

1. When a person is arrested on a charge of committing an offence of rape or an attempt to commit rape and there are reasonable grounds for believing that an examination of his person will afford evidence as to the commission of such offence, it shall be lawful for a RMP employed in a hospital run by the Government or by a local authority and in the absence of such a practitioner within the radius of 16 kilometers from the place where the offence has been committed by any other RMP, acting at the request of a police officer not below the rank of a Sub-Inspector, and for any person acting in good faith in his aid and under his direction, to make such an examination of the arrested person and to use such force as is reasonably necessary for that purpose.
2. The RMP conducting such examination shall, without delay, examine such person and prepare a report of his/her examination giving the following particulars, namely:
    a. The name and address of the accused and of the person by whom he was brought
    b. The age of the accused, marks of injury, if any, on the person of the accused
    d. The description of material taken from the person of the accused for DNA profiling
    e. Other material particulars in reasonable detail.
3. The report shall state precisely the reasons for each conclusion arrived at.
4. The exact time of commencement and completion of the examination shall also be noted in the report.
5. The RMP shall, without delay, forward the report of the investigating officer, who shall forward it to the Magistrate.

Table 4.1: Drafting of opinion based on examination findings and FSL report.

Genital injuries	Physical injuries	Provisional opinion	FSL report	Final opinion
Present	Present	There are signs suggestive of recent forceful penetration of vagina/anus. Opinion regarding intercourse is reserved till FSL report is received.	Positive for presence of semen	There are signs suggestive of recent forceful vaginal/anal intercourse.
			Negative for presence of semen/lubricant	There are no signs suggestive vaginal/anal intercourse, but evidence of physical and genital assault present.
Present	Absent	There are signs suggestive of recent forceful penetration of vagina/anus.	Positive for presence of semen	There are signs suggestive of recent forceful vaginal/anal intercourse.
			Negative for presence of semen/lubricant	There are no signs suggestive of recent vaginal/anal intercourse, but there is evidence of genital assault.
Absent	Present	There are signs of use of force, however, final opinion is reserved pending availability of FSL reports.	Positive for semen	There are signs suggestive of forceful vaginal/anal intercourse.
			Negative for semen/lubricant	There are no signs suggestive of vaginal/anal intercourse, but there is evidence of physical assault.
Absent	Absent	There are no signs of use of force; however final opinion is reserved pending availability of FSL reports.	Positive for semen	There are signs suggestive of vaginal/anal intercourse.
			Positive for semen and alcohol	There are signs suggestive of vaginal/anal intercourse under the influence of alcohol.
			Positive for lubricant	There is a possibility of vaginal/anal penetration by lubricated object.
			Negative for semen/alcohol/ lubricant	There are no signs suggestive of vaginal/anal intercourse or penetration of vagina/anus.

(FSL: Forensic science laboratory)

EX. 4.1: EXAMINATION OF SURVIVOR OF SEXUAL ASSAULT

FM 14.14: To examine and prepare medico-legal report of a survivor/victim of sexual offence in a simulated/supervised environment.

Chandrika Khobragade, a 16-year-old girl was brought by the police with alleged history of sexual assault by her neighbor. She was sexually assaulted in the fields when she had gone there to attend nature's call. She is thin built, 154 cm tall and weighed 48 kg. The victim presented with torn garments at places, stained with mud and sand particles, and stated that she has been raped at knife-point. The incident happened between 8.00 to 9.00 PM and she was brought to the emergency by the constable for examination at 11 PM on the same day. Prepare a medico-legal report for the same.

Department of Forensic Medicine and Toxicology

MLR No. ________________   CR. No. ________________

Patient Details

Name ____ D/W/S of ________________________________

Address ____

Age (as reported) __________ years   Date of birth (if known) ________________

Gender ____________________   Marital status: Unmarried/Married/Divorced

Occupation ____________________________ Educational status ________________________________

Contact phone no. (if any) ____

Examination Details

Date and Time of arrival in the hospital ________________________________

Date and Time of commencement of examination____

Brought by (Name and signatures)

a. If police: Name ____________________ P.C. No.________________ P.S.________________________

b. If not brought by police, name and relation with the examinee ________________________________

Any identified special needs/mental health problems ____

(Interpreters or special educators will be needed where the survivor has special needs such as hearing/speech disability, language barriers, intellectual or psychosocial disability)

Name of Social worker/Care worker (if any) ____

Informed Consent

I, ____ D/W/S of ____

hereby voluntary consent and agree to the following: *(Tick '✓')*

☐ Medical examination for treatment
☐ Medico-legal examination
☐ Sample collection for clinical and forensic examination

I understand that the medico-legal examination will include:
- A full medical history and complete examination (including examination of genital organs);
- Collection of forensic and medical specimens;
- Taking of notes, photographs/digital images for recording and evidential purposes;
- I understand and agree that a copy of the medical notes may be given to professionals involved in the case (e.g., police or lawyers) and may be used in the court;
- I agree to the use of my anonymized photographs/digital images/medical notes for teaching, audit and research;
- I have been informed that I may halt the examination at anytime with possible consequences of such refusal viz. loss of evidence and documentation. I have been further informed that this refusal will not effect my medical treatment.
- I also understand that as per law the hospital is required to inform police and this has been explained to me.

I want the information to be revealed to the police ☐ Yes ☐ No

The above have been explained to me in ____ language with the help of a

special educator/interpreter/support person *(circle as appropriate)*.

Date____________

Name and signature (thumb impression) of survivor
(Parents/guardian/person in whom the child reposes
trust in case of child < 12 years)

Signature and name of witness along with date and time ____

Signature and name of special educator/interpreter has ____

Signature and name of female nurse/attendant (in case of male doctor) ____

Marks of Identification

1. ____

2. ____

Brief history of assault (use separate sheet, if necessary) ____

____

____

____

Narrator of the incident (specify name and relation to survivor, if not self) ____

Details of Assailant(s)

Number of assailants and name/(s) ____

Sex of assailant(s) ____________________   Age of assailant(s) __________________

Prior knowledge of assailant(s) (relationship with the survivor) _______________________________

Last contact with alleged assailant(s) ____

Medical History

General health ____

Pre-existing skin problems, e.g., eczema, lichen sclerosus ________________________________

Previous illnesses ____

Operations ____

Menstrual/Obstetric History

Age of menarche __________ years/Not attained/Menopause attained

Periods (e.g., frequency/regularity/LMP) ____

Pre-existing menstrual problems, e.g., intermenstrual and postcoital bleeding __________________________

Menstruation at the time of incident   ☐ Yes   ☐ No

Menstruation at the time of examination   ☐ Yes   ☐ No

Post assault, has there been any vaginal discharge/bleeding?   ☐ Yes   ☐ No

Prior assault, has there been any vaginal discharge/bleeding?   ☐ Yes   ☐ No

Was the survivor pregnant at time of incident?   ☐ Yes   ☐ No

       If yes, duration of pregnancy ________________ weeks

Any children __________________ Mode of delivery ____________ Episiotomy ________________

Medications and Allergies

Prescribed medication ____

Vaccination status: Tetanus (Vaccinated/Not vaccinated)

Hepatitis B (Vaccinated/Not vaccinated)

Allergies ____

DETAILS OF THE ASSAULT FROM EXAMINEE

Specific Information Relating to the Alleged Offence

Date and Time of assault _________________________________ Time interval to examination _________________

Type of surface where assault occurred ____

Whether sleeping or unconscious at the time of the incident? ____

Whether cried for help or struggled or resisted? ____

Query	Tick '✓'			Details
Kissing/licking/biting/sucking/ spitting *(sites)*	☐ Not Known	☐ No	☐ Yes	
Penile-oral penetration	☐ Not Known	☐ No	☐ Yes	
Digital penetration	☐ Not Known	☐ No	☐ Yes	
Penile-vaginal penetration	☐ Not Known	☐ No	☐ Yes	
Mouth to genitalia/anus	☐ Not Known	☐ No	☐ Yes	
Penile-anal penetration	☐ Not Known	☐ No	☐ Yes	
Object to vulva/vagina/anus	☐ Not Known	☐ No	☐ Yes	
Other sexual/physical act(s)	☐ Not Known	☐ No	☐ Yes	
Ejaculation onto skin/hair	☐ Not Known	☐ No	☐ Yes	
Condom used throughout	☐ Not Known	☐ No	☐ Yes	
Lubricant/spermicide used	☐ Not Known	☐ No	☐ Yes	
Injuries	☐ Not Known	☐ No	☐ Yes	
Anogenital bleeding	☐ Not Known	☐ No	☐ Yes	
Damage to clothing	☐ Not Known	☐ No	☐ Yes	

Threat Used During Assault

a. Physical violence *(Tick '✓')*

☐ Hit with hand, fist, blunt object, sharp object	☐ Bitten	☐ Pulled hair
☐ Burned	☐ Kicked	☐ Pinched
☐ Violently shaken	☐ Head banged	☐ Dragged

b. Emotional abuse (insulting, cursing, belittling, terrorizing) ____

c. Use of restraints, if any ____

d. Used or threatened the use of weapon(s) or objects, if any____

e. Verbal threats (e.g., threats of killing or hurting survivor or any other person in whom the survivor is interested; use of photographs for blackmailing, etc.), if any:____

f. Luring (sweets, chocolates, money or job), if any: ____

g. Any other ____

If survivor has left any marks of injury on assailant/s (details) ____

Aggravating factors, e.g., injuries in contact with assailant's blood or semen   ☐ No   ☐ Yes

Post Assault (*Ask if relevant*)

☐ Brushed teeth/gums/dentures   ☐ Mouthwash/spray used

☐ Washed/bathed/douched   ☐ Changed tampon/pad/sponge/diaphragm

Oral intercourse: Drank/eaten food	☐ Not Known ☐ No ☐ Yes
Anal intercourse: Defecated since offence	☐ Not Known ☐ No ☐ Yes
Genital/anal/relevant skin: Wiped/washed Specify site and disposal of cloth/tissue	☐ Not Known ☐ No ☐ Yes ______________________
Passed urine	☐ Not Known ☐ No ☐ Yes (note time)
Changed/washed clothes If changed, are the clothes available?	☐ Not Known ☐ No ☐ Yes ☐ No ☐ Yes
Cleaned/washed undergarments	☐ Not Known ☐ No ☐ Yes
Self-harm	(sites)

Direct Questions (*Ask if relevant*)

Complaint	Since assault	Details (If yes, note if this was previously experienced)
Abdominal pain		
Urinary symptoms (e.g., dysuria, frequency, hematuria, incontinence, UTI)		
Genital symptoms (e.g., soreness, discharge, bleeding, dysperunia, pruritis, injuries)		
Bowel symptoms (e.g., soreness, pain on defecation, dyspareunia, bleeding, change in bowel habit, incontinence, pruritis, injuries)		

Sexual History

Dates and times of consensual sexual activity within the previous 10 days ________________________________

Items used in previous intercourse

Condom   ☐ Not Known   ☐ No   ☐ Yes

Spermicide   ☐ Not Known   ☐ No   ☐ Yes

Lubricant   ☐ Not Known   ☐ No   ☐ Yes

If relevant, clarify types of intercourse in last 10 days only: ________________________________

Drug and Alcohol use in Relation to Assault

Was alcohol consumed? ☐ Not Known ☐ No ☐ Yes

If yes, please specify ☐ Post Offence ☐ Prior ☐ During

Start time of drinking _________________________ End time of drinking _________________________

Quantity and type of beverage consumed ____

Time last ate ____

Any illicit drugs been used/administered to the ☐ Not Known ☐ No ☐ Yes
survivor within 4 days of the examination?

If yes, please specify ☐ Post Offence ☐ Prior ☐ During

Give details ____

Are any other substances having been used/ ☐ Not Known ☐ No ☐ Yes
administered that could be relevant to the offence?

If yes, please specify ☐ Post Offence ☐ Prior ☐ During

Give details ____

General Examination

Clothes

- Condition of clothes: Tears/cuts/rents/burnt
- Foreign matter/Stains: Blood/seminal/fecal/mud/grass/any other_________________________
- Buttons: Intact/undone/broken/torn

Built: Well/Average/Poor

Height _______ cm Weight _________ kg

Pulse ________/min BP __________ mm Hg Respiratory rate ________/min

Conscious level ____

General appearance ____

Skin (color, gooseflesh, etc.) ____

Hair (hair style, last wash, any added hair dye) ____

Demeanor/behavior ☐ Sober ☐ Eccentric ☐ Erratic ☐ Calm ☐ Depressed

Speech (e.g., content, form) ____

Pre-existing physical problems (note type) ____

Secondary sexual characters ____

Injuries (Type, site, size, shape, color, swelling and signs of healing)

Site Examined		Injuries	Type of injury	Features/Remarks
Scalp		☐ No ☐ Yes		
Face		☐ No ☐ Yes		
Eyes		☐ No ☐ Yes		
Ears		☐ No ☐ Yes		
Lips		☐ No ☐ Yes		
Inside mouth/palate		☐ No ☐ Yes		
Teeth		☐ No ☐ Yes		
Neck		☐ No ☐ Yes		
Back		☐ No ☐ Yes		
Buttocks		☐ No ☐ Yes		
Arms	Right	☐ No ☐ Yes		
	Left	☐ No ☐ Yes		
Hands/wrists	Right	☐ No ☐ Yes		
	Left	☐ No ☐ Yes		
Fingers/nails	Right	☐ No ☐ Yes		
	Left	☐ No ☐ Yes		
Breasts		☐ No ☐ Yes		
Abdomen		☐ No ☐ Yes		
Legs	Right	☐ No ☐ Yes		
	Left	☐ No ☐ Yes		
Feet/ankles/soles				
	Right	☐ No ☐ Yes		
	Left	☐ No ☐ Yes		
Additional details (injection sites, self-harm, etc.)				

(Tick '✓')

Systemic Examination

Cardiorespiratory System

Heart sounds, Trachea/air entry, breath sounds _______________________________

____

Abdomen

Liver, Kidneys, Spleen ____

Tenderness/masses ____

Bowel sounds ____

Central Nervous Systems

Pupil size and reactions ____

Eye movement/nystagmus ____

Conjunctivae ____

Balance/coordination ____

Reflexes ______________________________ Tremor _____________________________

Genital and Anal Examination

Details of Female Genital Findings

Site Examined	Findings *(Bleeding/tear/discharge/edema/tenderness)*
Thighs	
Mons pubis, perineal tear	
Pubic hair (matted, shaved, cut)	
Labia majora	
Labia minora	
Clitoris	
Fourchette	
Fossa navicularis	
Vestibule	
Urethra	
Hymen (edges, position of tear)	
Posterior commissure	

Internal findings (if applicable)

Vaginal wall ____

Cervix ____

Details of Anal Findings

Natal fold	
Perianal/anal margin	
Internal findings	

Specific Examinations *(wherever facilities exists, and if indicated)*

a. Toluidine blue dye test ____

b. Per speculum findings, if performed* _________________________________

c. Per vaginum findings, if performed* __________________________________

d. Wet mount slide test ____

e. UV light examination of clothes and skin _____________________________

f. Colposcopic/Proctoscopic examination ________________________________

* Per vaginum/per speculum examination *should not be done* unless required for detection of injuries or for medical treatment.

Details of Male Genital Findings

Site	Findings *(Bleeding/tear/discharge/edema/tenderness)*
Thighs	
Pubic area	
Pubic hair	
Scrotum	
Testes	
Penis	
Foreskin	

Sample Collected/Investigations for Hospital/Clinical Laboratory

(Tick '✓')

☐ Blood for HIV, VDRL, HbsAg

☐ Urine test for pregnancy

☐ Ultrasound for pregnancy/internal injury

☐ X-ray/CT for injury

Samples Collected for Forensic Science Laboratory

(Samples to be packed, sealed and labeled separately. Swab sticks should be moistened with distilled water)

1. Debris collection paper

2. Clothing evidence where available (to be packed in separate paper bags after air drying)

Body evidence samples, as appropriate (duly labeled and packed separately)*

Samples	Collected/Not collected	Reason(s) for not collecting
Swabs from stains on the body		
Scalp hair (10–15 strands)		
Head hair combing		
Nail scrapings/clippings (both hands)		
Oral swab		
Blood for grouping (plain vial)		
Blood for drug/alcohol levels (sodium fluoride vial)		
Blood for DNA analysis (EDTA vial/FTA card)		
Urine (drug testing)		
Any other (tampon/sanitary napkin/condom/object)		

*Genital and Anal Evidence**

Samples	Collected/Not collected	Reason(s) for not collecting
Matted pubic hair		
Pubic hair combing and cutting (mention, if shaved)		
Two vulval swabs (for semen and DNA testing)		
Two vaginal swabs (for semen and DNA testing)		
Two anal swabs (for semen and DNA testing)		
Vaginal smear (air-dried) for semen examination		
Vaginal washing		
Urethral swab		
Swab from clitoris/glans of penis		

*Samples to be preserved in refrigerator till handed over to police along with duly attested sample seal.

Treatment prescribed ____

Time of completion of examination ____

Provisional Medical Opinion

I have examined (name of survivor) ____ aged about ___________ years

reporting with alleged history of (type of sexual violence and circumstances) ___________________________________

____ after ___________________ (days/hours) of the

incident. My findings are as follows:
- Important clinical findings ____
- Additional observations (if any) ____
- Samples collected (for FSL), awaiting reports ____
- Samples collected (for hospital laboratory)____

On the basis of above mentioned observations, I am of the opinion that *(Refer to Table 4.1)* ___________________

____

____

Place ________________   ___________________________
                                                          Signature of the Doctor
Date ________________   Name, Designation and Seal

Copy of the Entire Medical Report must be Given to the Survivor Free of Cost Immediately

This report contains ……………………....................…….. number of sheets and ……………………....................……….. number of envelopes and ……………………...................…….. number of samples.

____

Received MLR No. _____________________ along with body diagram and _________________ number of envelopes, _____________ number of samples and sample seal.

Name _______________________________________ P.C. No. _____________________ P.S. _______________

                                                          ____
                                                          Signature and Date

Date _________

MLR No. _________

CR No. _________

____

Signature of the Doctor
Name, Designation and Seal

EX. 4.1A: FINAL OPINION REGARDING SURVIVOR/VICTIM OF SEXUAL VIOLENCE

FM 14.14: Demonstrate an understanding of framing the opinion in such cases.

Department of Forensic Medicine and Toxicology

____

To   Date ______________

The Investigating Officer,

_____________________ Police Station

_____________________ (District/City/Town)

Ref:

a.   FSL report no. _____________________ dated __________

b.   Toxicology report no. ___________ dated __________

As per requisition from the ___________________________________ of ___________________________

police station dated __________________, medico-legal examination was conducted on ___________________

D/W of _________________________________ aged about __________________ years, gender ______________,

and the MLR number _________________ dated _______________________ was issued by the undersigned.

Taking into account the history, clinical examination findings and FSL reports, I am of the opinion that: _(Refer to Table 4.1)_

____
Signature of the Doctor
Name, Designation and Seal

Place __________

Date __________

____

Received final opinion regarding MLR No. ______________ dated __________.

Name ___________________________________ P.C. No. _________________________ P.S. ________________

____
Signature and Date

EX. 4.2: EXAMINATION OF ACCUSED OF SEXUAL OFFENCE

FM 14.13: To examine and prepare report of an alleged accused person in cases of various sexual offences in a simulated/supervised environment.

Mukesh Singh, a 37-year-old male was brought by the police with alleged history of raping his neighbor. He is well built, 179 cm tall and weighed 78 kg. The incident took place 6.00 to 7.00 PM and the police arrested him from his friend's place at 12 midnight and brought him for examination. Prepare a medico-legal report for the same.

Department of Forensic Medicine and Toxicology

____

MLR No. ________________   C.R. No. ______________

Patient Details

Name ____ Son of_________________________________

Address ____

Age (as reported) ________ years   Date of birth (if known) __________________

Gender ___________________   Marital status: Unmarried/Married/Divorced

Examination Details

Date and Time of examination______________________________

Requisition from ______________________________ Vide letter no. ______________ Dated __________

Brought by (Name and signature) _______________________ P.C. No.______________ P.S.____________

Informed Consent

(Consent is asked for, but if refused, reasonable force may be used if examination is done under Sec. 53A CrPC)

I, ______________________________________Son of ______________________________________

hereby give my consent for examination and sample collection for medico-legal examination, knowing that the result of the examination may go in my favor or against.

I understand that the examination will include:
- A full medical history and complete examination (including examination of genital organs);
- Collection of forensic specimens;
- Taking of photographs/digital images for recording and evidential purposes;
- I understand and agree that a copy of the medical notes may be given to professionals involved in the case (e.g., police or lawyers) and may be used in the court;
- I agree to the use of my anonymized photographs/digital images/medical notes for teaching, audit and research.

The above have been explained to me in _______________________________ language which I can understand.

Date____________

Name and signature (thumb impression)
of the examinee

Marks of Identification

1. ____

2. ____

Brief history of assault as stated by the accused (use separate sheet, if necessary) _______________

____

____

____

Did the accused know the victim before? ☐ No ☐ Yes If yes, relationship _______________

Medical History and Allergies

General health ____

Pre-existing skin problems, e.g., eczema, lichen sclerosus ____

Prescribed medication ____

Vaccination status: Hepatitis B (Vaccinated/Not vaccinated)

Allergies ____

DETAILS OF THE ASSAULT FROM EXAMINEE

Specific Information Relating to the Alleged Offence

Date and time of assault _____________________________ Time interval to examination _______________

Type of surface where assault occurred ____

Query	Tick '✓'			Details
Kissing/licking/biting/sucking/ spitting (*sites*)	☐ Not Known	☐ No	☐ Yes	
Penile-oral penetration	☐ Not Known	☐ No	☐ Yes	
Penile-anal penetration	☐ Not Known	☐ No	☐ Yes	
Penile-vaginal penetration	☐ Not Known	☐ No	☐ Yes	
Digital penetration	☐ Not Known	☐ No	☐ Yes	
Mouth to genitalia/anus	☐ Not Known	☐ No	☐ Yes	
Object to vulva/vagina/anus	☐ Not Known	☐ No	☐ Yes	
Other sexual/physical act(s)	☐ Not Known	☐ No	☐ Yes	
Ejaculation onto skin/hair	☐ Not Known	☐ No	☐ Yes	
Condom used throughout	☐ Not Known	☐ No	☐ Yes	
Lubricant/spermicide used	☐ Not Known	☐ No	☐ Yes	
Injuries inflicted	☐ Not Known	☐ No	☐ Yes	
Damage to clothing	☐ Not Known	☐ No	☐ Yes	

Threat Used During Assault

a. Physical violence *(Tick '✓')*

☐ Hit with hand, fist, blunt object, sharp object	☐ Bitten	☐ Pulled hair
☐ Burned	☐ Kicked	☐ Pinched
☐ Violently shaken	☐ Head banged	☐ Dragged

b. Emotional abuse (insulting, cursing, belittling, terrorizing) _______________________

c. Use of restraints, if any ____

d. Used weapon(s) or objects, if any ____

e. Verbal threats, if any:____

f. Luring (sweets, chocolates, money or job), if any: __________________________________

g. Any other ____

If survivor has injured the accused (details) ____

Post Assault

Genital/relevant skin: Wiped/washed Specify site and disposal of cloth/tissue	☐ Not Known ☐ No ☐ Yes _______________________________________
Passed urine	☐ Not Known ☐ No ☐ Yes (note time)
Oral intercourse: Drank/eaten food	☐ Not Known ☐ No ☐ Yes
Anal intercourse: Defecated since offence	☐ Not Known ☐ No ☐ Yes
Changed/washed clothes If changed, are the clothes available?	☐ Not Known ☐ No ☐ Yes ☐ No ☐ Yes
Cleaned/washed undergarments	☐ Not Known ☐ No ☐ Yes
Taken bath/shower	☐ Not Known ☐ No ☐ Yes

Drug and Alcohol use in Relation to Assault

Was alcohol consumed?   ☐ Not Known   ☐ No   ☐ Yes

If yes, please specify   ☐ Post Offence   ☐ Prior   ☐ During

Start time of drinking ____________________ End time of drinking ____________________

Quantity and type of beverage consumed ____

Any illicit drugs been used within 4 days of the examination?   ☐ Not Known   ☐ No   ☐ Yes

If yes, specify   ☐ Post Offence   ☐ Prior   ☐ During

Give details ____

General Examination

Clothes

- Foreign matter/Stains: Blood/seminal/fecal/mud/lipstick/hair/grass/any other _______________________

- Buttons/zipper: Intact/undone/broken/torn

Built: Well/Average/Poor   Height _______ cm   Weight _______ kg

Pulse _______/min   BP __________ mm Hg   Respiratory rate ______/min

General appearance ____

Signs of intoxication ____

Demeanor/behavior   ☐ Sober   ☐ Excited   ☐ Terrified   ☐ Calm   ☐ Depressed

Speech (e.g., content, form) ____

Secondary sexual characters ____

Injuries (type, site, size, shape, color, swelling and signs of healing)/Scar/Stains/Foreign body

Site Examined		Injuries	Type of injury	Features/Remarks
Face		☐ No ☐ Yes		
Eyes		☐ No ☐ Yes		
Lips		☐ No ☐ Yes		
Teeth		☐ No ☐ Yes		
Neck		☐ No ☐ Yes		
Back		☐ No ☐ Yes		
Arms	Right Left	☐ No ☐ Yes ☐ No ☐ Yes		
Hands/wrists	Right Left	☐ No ☐ Yes ☐ No ☐ Yes		
Fingers/nails	Right Left	☐ No ☐ Yes ☐ No ☐ Yes		
Front of chest		☐ No ☐ Yes		
Abdomen		☐ No ☐ Yes		
Additional details				

(Tick '✓')

Systemic Examination ____

Genital Examination

General development ____

Site Examined	Findings *(stains/foreign body/bleeding/tear/edema/tenderness)*
Thighs	
Pubic area	
Pubic hair (matted/shaved/cut)	
Scrotum	
Testes	
Prepuce	Retractable/Nonretractable/Circumcised
Smegma (retract prepuce and observe)	Present/Absent
Frenulum	Torn/Intact
Penis (any deformity, abrasion, smell)	
Signs of sexually transmitted disease (discharge)	

Specific Examination *(if done)*

Lugol's iodine test ____

Sample Collected/Investigations for Hospital Laboratory

1. Blood for HIV, VDRL, HbsAg, WR and Kahn test
2. X-ray/CT for injury

Samples Collected for Forensic Science Laboratory

(Samples to be packed, sealed and labeled separately. Swab sticks should be moistened with distilled water)

1. Debris collection paper
2. Clothing evidence, where available (to be packed in separate paper bags after air drying)

Body Evidence Samples, as Appropriate (Duly Labeled and Packed Separately)*

Samples	Collected/Not collected	Reason(s) for not collecting
Swabs from stains on the body/teeth bite		
Scalp hair (10–15 strands)		
Nail scrapings/clippings (both hands)		
Blood for grouping (plain vial)		
Blood for drug/alcohol levels (sodium fluoride vial)		
Blood for DNA analysis (EDTA vial/FTA card)		
Urine (drug testing)		
Any other (e.g., swab from discharge, lubricant)		

*Genital Evidence**

Samples	Collected/Not collected	Reason(s) for not collecting
Matted pubic hair		
Pubic hair combing and cutting (mention, if shaved)		
Prostatic swab for gonorrheal secretions		
Swab from prepuce, coronal sulcus (vaginal cells/fecal matter)		

*Samples to be preserved in refrigerator till handed over to police along with duly attested sample seal.

Time of completion of examination _______________________________

Provisional Medical Opinion

Taking into consideration the history of the case and clinical examination, I am of the opinion that:

☐ The possibility of recent performance of sexual intercourse cannot be ruled out, i.e., there is evidence of recent penetration of vagina/anus. However, final opinion will be given after receiving the FSL report.

☐ The examinee is incapable of performing sexual intercourse in the ordinary way or accomplish penetration (gross penile deformity).
(*Tick '✓'*)

Place ________________

Date ________________

Signature of the Doctor

Name, Designation and Seal

Received MLR No. ___________ along with body diagram and ___________ number of envelopes, ___________ number of samples and sample seal.

Name ____ P.C. No. _____________________ P.S. ________________

Signature and Date

Date ___________   **MLR No.** ___________   **CR No.** ___________

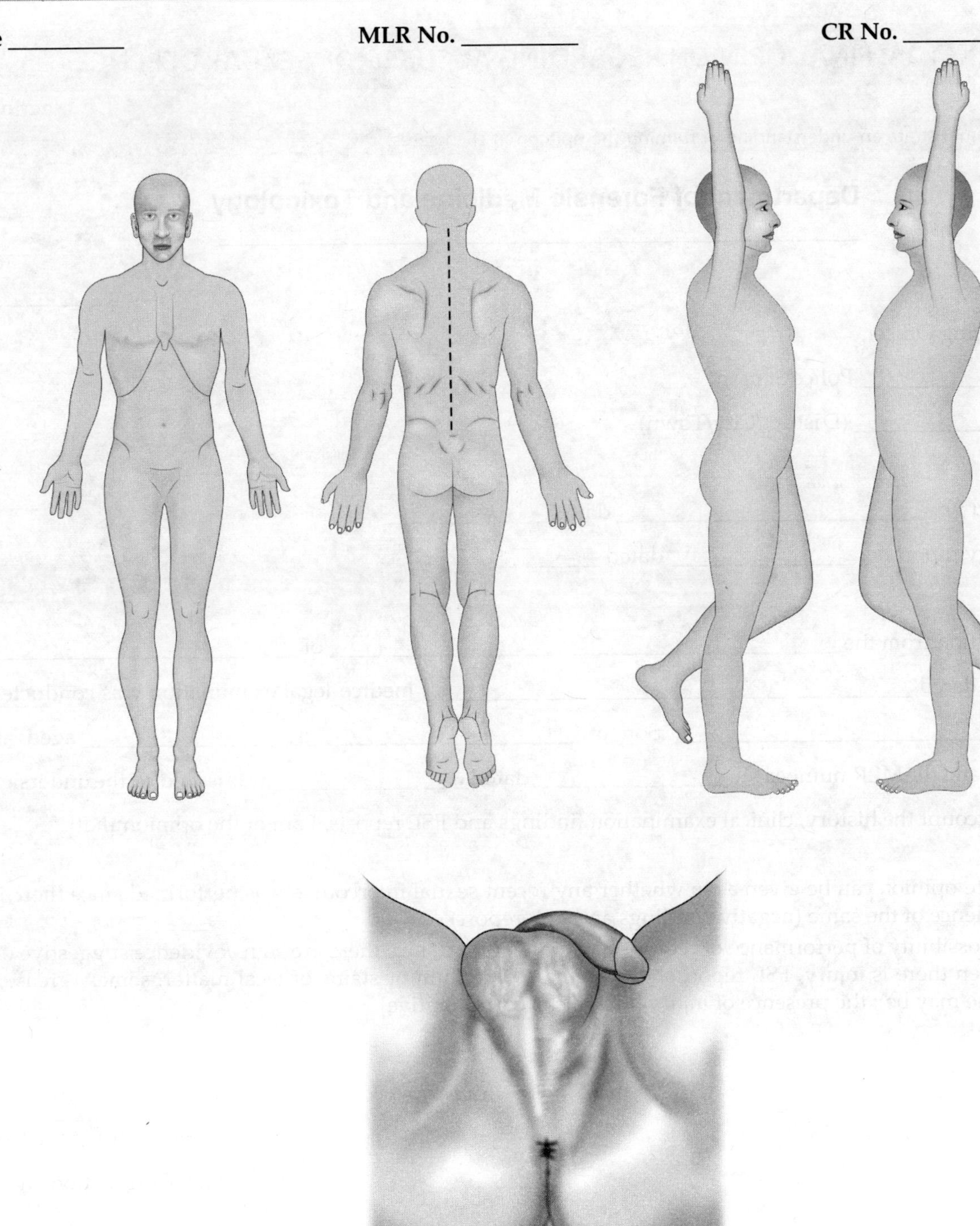

____

Signature of the Doctor
Name, Designation and Seal

EX. 4.2A: FINAL OPINION REGARDING ACCUSED OF SEXUAL OFFENCE

FM 14.13: Demonstrate an understanding of framing the opinion in such cases.

Department of Forensic Medicine and Toxicology

To

Date ______________

The Investigating Officer,

______________________Police Station

______________________ (District/City/Town)

Ref:

a. FSL report no. ______________________ dated ______________

b. Toxicology report no. ______________ dated __________

As per requisition from the ____ of ______________________________

police station dated ____, medico-legal examination was conducted on

____ Son of ____ aged about

________ years and the MLR number ______________________ dated ________________ was issued by the undersigned.

Taking into account the history, clinical examination findings and FSL reports, I am of the opinion that:

☐ No definite opinion can be given as to whether any recent sexual intercourse was performed since there is no signs/evidence of the same (negative findings and FSL report)

☐ There is possibility of performance of recent sexual intercourse since there are signs/evidence suggestive of the same [when there is injury, FSL report show vaginal epithelium or stains of fecal matter, semen, grease, etc. (as the case may be); the presence of injury on penis is corroborative]
(Tick '✓')

____

Signature of the Doctor

Place ______________________

Name, Designation and Seal

Date ______________________

Received final opinion regarding MLR No. ______________________ dated ____ .

Name______________________________________P.C.No.______________________P.S.______________________

____

Signature and Date

EX. 4.3: EXAMINATION OF VICTIM OF FORCED/NON-CONSENSUAL PENETRATIVE ANAL SEX

FM 14.14: To examine and prepare medico-legal report of a survivor/victim of various sexual offences (forced/non-consensual penetrative anal sex) in a simulated/supervised environment.

Manish Ranawat, a 13-year-old boy was allegedly sodomized by his acquaintance after luring him to a lonely spot while they were playing cricket. There the accused forcefully had sex and later forced him to clean up. He also threatened the victim with death threats and to keep quiet about the act. His parents complained to the police who brought the victim for examination. Prepare a report for the same.

Department of Forensic Medicine and Toxicology

MLR No. _________________   C.R. No. _______________

Patient Details

Name _______________________________________ S/D/W of _______________________________

Address ____

Age (as reported) _______ years   Date of birth (if known) _______________

Gender_____________________   Marital status: Unmarried/Married/Divorced

Examination Details

Date and Time of examination_______________________

Requisition from _________________________________ Vide letter no. _______________ Dated ___________

Brought by (Name and signature) _______________________ P.C. No._______________ P.S._______________

Informed Consent

I, _________________________________ S/D/W of ____

hereby give my consent for examination and sample collection for medico-legal examination, knowing that the result of the examination may go in my favor or against.

I understand that the examination will include:
- A full medical history and complete examination (including examination of genital organs);
- Collection of forensic specimens;
- Taking of photographs/digital images for recording and evidential purposes;
- I understand and agree that a copy of the medical notes may be given to professionals involved in the case (e.g., police or lawyers) and may be used in the court;
- I agree to the use of my anonymized photographs/digital images/medical notes for teaching, audit and research.

The above have been explained to me in _________________________________ language which I can understand.

Date_____________

Name and signature (thumb impression)
of the examinee

Marks of Identification

1. ____

2. ____

History

As given by police _______________________________________

Brief history of assault as stated by the accused (use separate sheet, if necessary) _______________

____

____

____

Did the accused know the victim before? ☐ No ☐ Yes If yes, relationship _______________

Medical History and Allergies

General health _______________________________________

Pre-existing skin problems, e.g., eczema, lichen sclerosus _______________

Prescribed medication _______________________________

Vaccination status: Hepatitis B (Vaccinated/Not vaccinated)

Allergies ____

DETAILS OF THE ASSAULT FROM EXAMINEE

Specific Information Relating to the Alleged Offence

Date and time of assault _______________________ Time interval to examination _______________

Whether sleeping or unconscious during the act? _______________________________

Whether cried for help or struggled or resisted? _______________________________

Query	Tick '✓'	Details
Kissing/licking/biting/sucking/ spitting *(sites)*	☐ Not Known ☐ No ☐ Yes	
Penile-oral penetration	☐ Not Known ☐ No ☐ Yes	
Penile-anal penetration	☐ Not Known ☐ No ☐ Yes	
Penile-vaginal penetration	☐ Not Known ☐ No ☐ Yes	
Digital penetration	☐ Not Known ☐ No ☐ Yes	
Mouth to genitalia/anus	☐ Not Known ☐ No ☐ Yes	
Object to vulva/vagina/anus	☐ Not Known ☐ No ☐ Yes	
Other sexual/physical act(s)	☐ Not Known ☐ No ☐ Yes	
Ejaculation onto skin/hair	☐ Not Known ☐ No ☐ Yes	

Condom used throughout	☐ Not Known	☐ No	☐ Yes	
Lubricant/spermicide used	☐ Not Known	☐ No	☐ Yes	
Injuries inflicted	☐ Not Known	☐ No	☐ Yes	
Damage to clothing	☐ Not Known	☐ No	☐ Yes	

Threat Used During Assault

a. Physical violence *(Tick '✓')*

☐ Hit with hand, fist, blunt object, sharp object	☐ Bitten	☐ Pulled hair
☐ Burned	☐ Kicked	☐ Pinched
☐ Violently shaken	☐ Head banged	☐ Dragged

b. Emotional abuse (insulting, cursing, belittling, terrorizing) ________________________

c. Use of restraints, if any ____

d. Used weapon(s) or objects, if any ____

e. Verbal threats, if any:____

f. Luring (sweets, chocolates, money or job), if any: ____________________________________

g. Any other ____

If survivor has injured the accused (details) ____

Post Assault

Genital/relevant skin: Wiped/washed Specify site and disposal of cloth/tissue	☐ Not Known ☐ No ☐ Yes ________________________________
Passed urine	☐ Not Known ☐ No ☐ Yes (note time)
Oral intercourse: Drank/eaten food	☐ Not Known ☐ No ☐ Yes
Anal intercourse: Defecated since offence	☐ Not Known ☐ No ☐ Yes
Changed/washed clothes If changed, are the clothes available?	☐ Not Known ☐ No ☐ Yes ☐ No ☐ Yes
Cleaned/washed undergarments	☐ Not Known ☐ No ☐ Yes
Taken bath/shower	☐ Not Known ☐ No ☐ Yes

Drug and Alcohol use in Relation to Assault

Was alcohol consumed? ☐ Not Known ☐ No ☐ Yes

If yes, please specify ☐ Post Offence ☐ Prior ☐ During

Start time of drinking ____________________________ End time of drinking ____________________

Quantity and type of beverage consumed ____

Any illicit drugs been used within 4 days of the examination? ☐ Not Known ☐ No ☐ Yes

If yes, specify ☐ Post Offence ☐ Prior ☐ During

Give details ____

General Examination

Clothes

- Foreign matter/Stains: Blood/seminal/fecal/mud/hair/grass/any other _______________________

- Buttons/zipper: Intact/undone/broken/torn

Built: Well/Average/Poor Height _______ cm Weight _______ kg

Pulse _______/min BP _______ mm Hg Respiratory rate _______/min

General appearance ____

Signs of intoxication ____

Demeanor/behavior ☐ Sober ☐ Excited ☐ Terrified ☐ Calm ☐ Depressed

Speech (e.g., content, form) ____

Secondary sexual characters ____

Injuries (type, site, size, shape, color, swelling and signs of healing)/Scar/Stains/Foreign body

Site Examined		Injuries		Type of injury	Features/Remarks
Face		☐ No	☐ Yes		
Eyes		☐ No	☐ Yes		
Lips		☐ No	☐ Yes		
Teeth		☐ No	☐ Yes		
Neck		☐ No	☐ Yes		
Back		☐ No	☐ Yes		
Arms	Right	☐ No	☐ Yes		
	Left	☐ No	☐ Yes		
Hands/wrists	Right	☐ No	☐ Yes		
	Left	☐ No	☐ Yes		
Fingers/nails	Right	☐ No	☐ Yes		
	Left	☐ No	☐ Yes		
Front of chest		☐ No	☐ Yes		
Abdomen		☐ No	☐ Yes		
Additional details					

(Tick '✓')

Systemic Examination ____

____

Genital Examination

General development ____

Site Examined	Findings *(stains/foreign body/bleeding/tear/edema/tenderness)*		
Thighs			
Pubic area			
Pubic hair (matted/shaved/cut)			
Signs of sexually transmitted disease			
Natal fold			
Perianal/anal margin			
Anus	Anal mucosa	☐ Smooth	☐ Thickened
	Tears	☐ Present	☐ Absent If present: Recent/Old
	Depression of anus	☐ Present	☐ Not present
	Hemorrhoids	☐ Present	☐ Not present
	Stains of blood/ semen/lubricants	☐ Present	☐ Absent
Anal sphincter	Tone	☐ Retained	☐ Lost
	Rugal pattern	☐ Retained	☐ Lost
	Lateral traction test	☐ Orifice closes	☐ Relaxes reflexly
	Per rectal	Admits one/more finger, with/without pain	
Rectum			

Speculum examination ____

Sample Collected/Investigations for Hospital Laboratory

1. Blood for HIV, VDRL, HbsAg
2. X-ray/CT for injury.

Samples Collected for Forensic Science Laboratory

(Samples to be packed, sealed and labeled separately. Swab sticks should be moistened with distilled water)

1. Debris collection paper
2. Clothing evidence, where available (to be packed in separate paper bags after air drying).

Body Evidence Samples, as Appropriate (Duly Labeled and Packed Separately)*

Samples	Collected/Not collected	Reason(s) for not collecting
Swabs from stains on the body/teeth bite		
Scalp hair (10–15 strands)		
Buccal swabs		
Nail scrapings/clippings (both hands)		
Blood for grouping (plain vial)		
Blood for drug/alcohol levels (sodium fluoride vial)		
Blood for DNA analysis (EDTA vial/FTA card)		
Urine (drug testing)		
Any other (e.g., swab from discharge, lubricant)		

*Genital Evidence**

Samples	Collected/Not collected	Reason(s) for not collecting
Matted pubic hair		
Pubic hair combing and cutting (mention, if shaved)		
Anal swabs		
Loose hair from anal region and buttocks		

*Samples to be preserved in refrigerator till handed over to police along with duly attested sample seal.

Time of completion of examination ___________________________________.

Provisional Medical Opinion

On the basis of above mentioned observations, I am of the opinion that the findings of examination is consistent with/not inconsistent with the history of alleged sexual intercourse, i.e., there is evidence of/no evidence of recent penetration of anus/buccal coitus. However, final opinion will be given after receiving of FSL report.

Place _______________

Date _______________

____
Signature of the Doctor

Name, Designation and Seal

Received MLR no. __________________ along with body diagram and ________________ number of envelopes,

________________ number of samples and sample seal.

Name ___________________________________ P.C. No. ____________________ P.S. ________________

____
Signature and Date

Date __________   **MLR No.** __________   **CR No.** __________

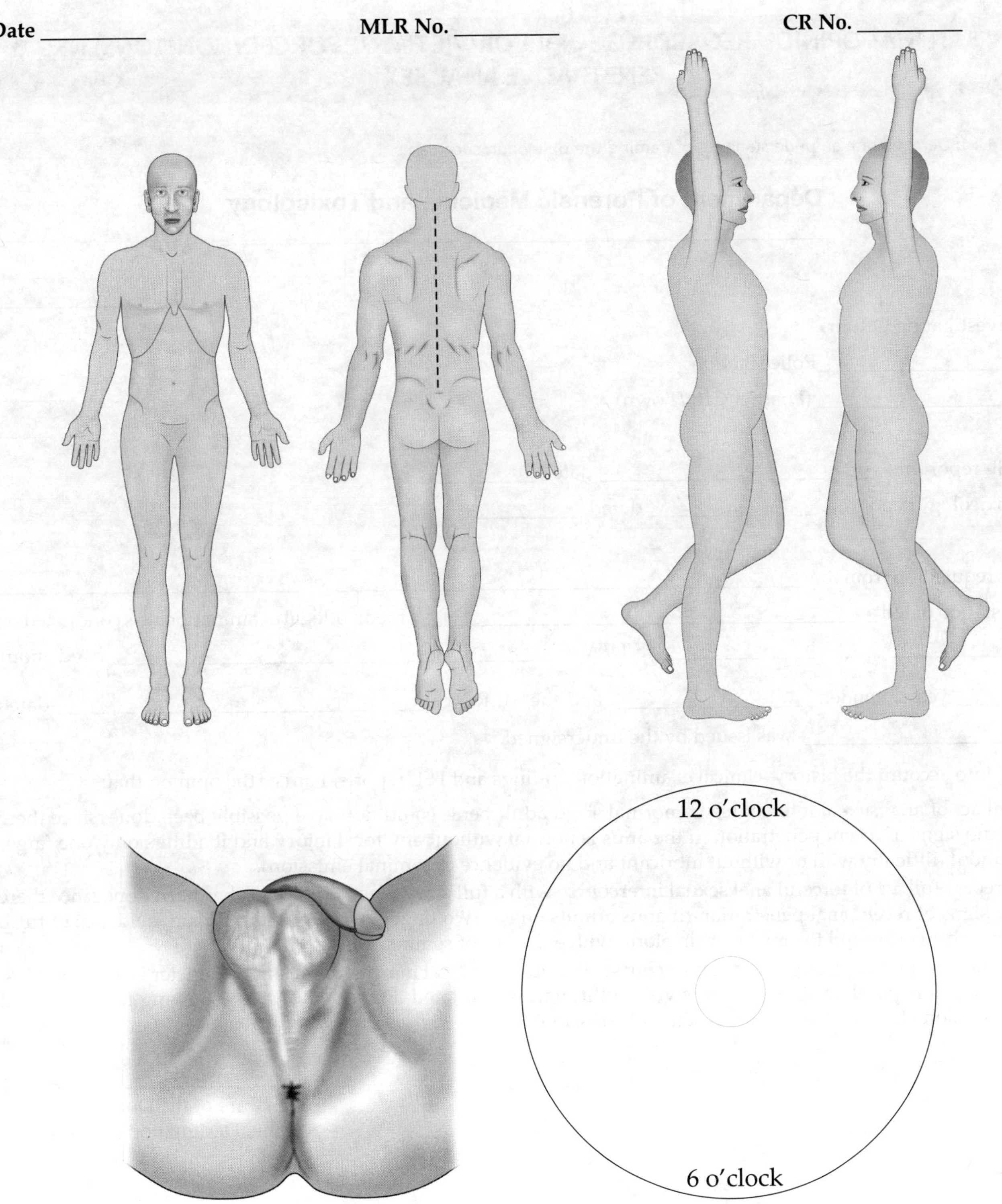

Signature of the Doctor
Name, Designation and Seal

EX. 4.3A: FINAL OPINION REGARDING SURVIVOR/VICTIM OF FORCED/NON-CONSENSUAL PENETRATIVE ANAL SEX

FM 14.14: Demonstrate an understanding of framing the opinion in such cases.

Department of Forensic Medicine and Toxicology

To

Date ____________

The Investigating Officer,

____________________Police Station

____________________ (District/City/Town)

Ref:

a.   FSL report no. ____________________ dated ____________

b.   Toxicology report no. ______________ dated __________

As per requisition from the ____ of ________________________________

police station dated ____, medico-legal examination was conducted on

____ S/D/W of ____ aged about

____________ years, gender __________________, and the MLR No. ________________________________ dated

________________________________ was issued by the undersigned.

Taking into account the history, clinical examination findings and FSL reports, I am of the opinion that:

☐   Full act of anal sexual intercourse by normal sized adult penis could not have possibly been done, since there are no signs of recent penetration (if the anus is normal without any focal injury and it admits only one finger without difficulty with or without lubricant and no evidence of seminal emission).

☐   A recent full act of forceful anal sexual intercourse with a full sized erect adult penis has been done since there are signs of recent anal penetration (if anus admits one or two fingers with or without pain, evidence of fresh tear or bruise around the anal margin along with evidence of seminal emission).

☐   There are signs suggestive of anal intercourse (if there is no focal injury but the anal sphincter is loose and lax, anal canal is patulous and rectum is visible through well dilated anal canal or anus showing funnel shaped depression along with evidence of seminal emission).
(Tick '✓')

____
Signature of the Doctor
Name, Designation and Seal

Place ________________

Date ________________

____

Received final opinion regarding MLR No. ________________________ dated ____________

Name ____________________________ P.C. No. ________________________________ P.S. ____________________

____
Signature and Date

EX. 4.4: COMMUNICATION WITH SURVIVOR AND ACCUSED OF SEXUAL ASSAULT

FM 14.13: Describe and discuss personal opinions and their impact on examination of accused and the need for objectivity/ neutrality to avoid prejudices influencing the case.
FM 14.14: Describe and discuss sympathetic/empathetic examination and interview of survivors/victims of sexual assault including presence of trusted figure in cases of minor victims.

PSYCHOSOCIAL CARE

Establishing Rapport with the Survivor ____

____

____

____

Addressing Survivor's Emotional Wellbeing ____

____

____

____

Creating and enabling Atmosphere and establishing Trust _________________________________

____

____

____

Role of Family, Friends and Community ____

____

____

____

In situations of Child abuse ____

____

____

____

Dealing with Adolescents Survivors ____

____

____

____

When Perpetrator of sexual assault is Parent/Guardian ___________________________________

____

____

CULTURAL AND SPIRITUAL ASPECTS

Survivor or accused from LGBTQIA+ ____

____

____

____

Sex worker ____

____

____

____

Caste and religion ____

____

____

____

EX. 4.5: COLLECTION AND PRESERVATION OF TRACE EVIDENCES

FM 14.13 and 14.14: Demonstrate understanding of preservation and dispatch of trace evidences from survivor and accused of sexual assault cases.

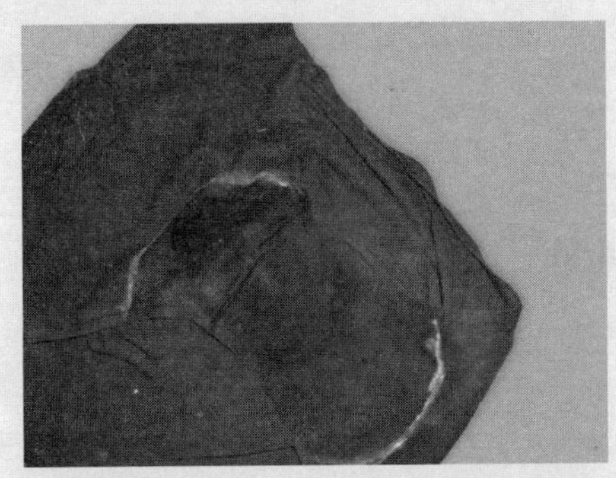	**Clothing**
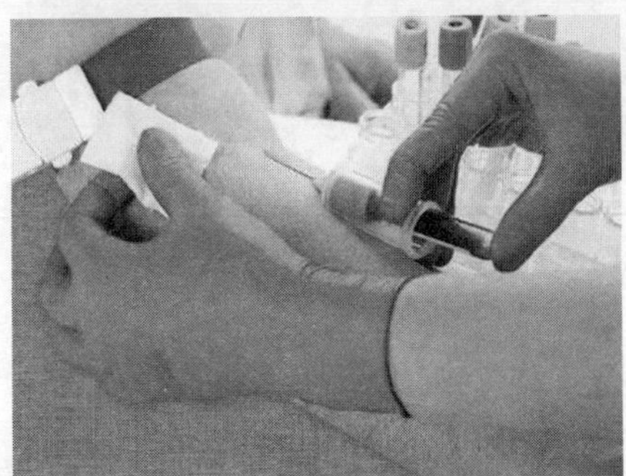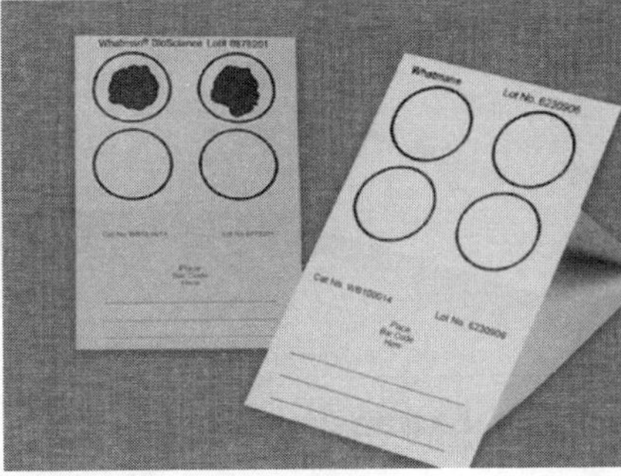	**DNA (Blood)**
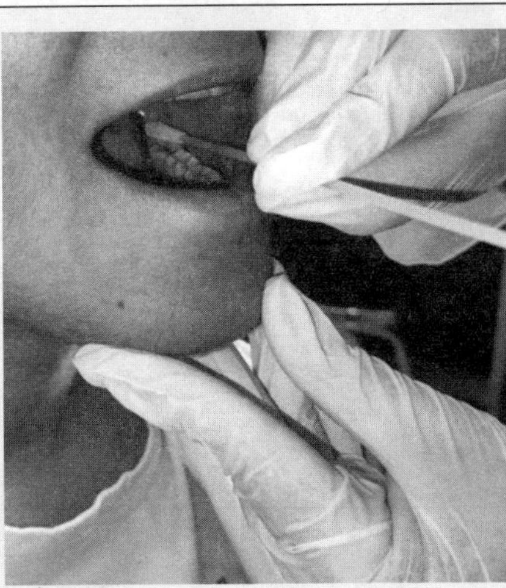	**Oral swabs**

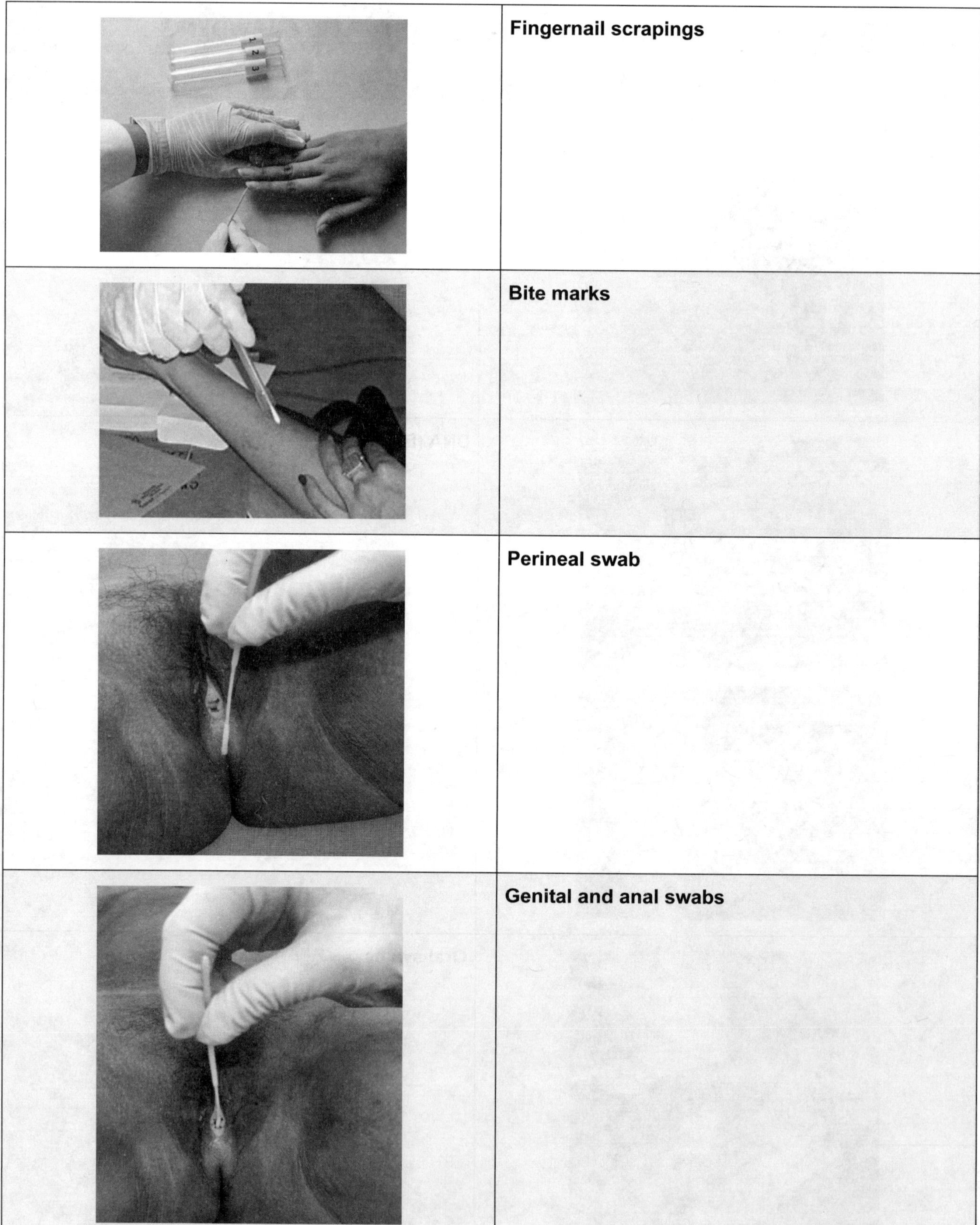

	Fingernail scrapings
	Bite marks
	Perineal swab
	Genital and anal swabs

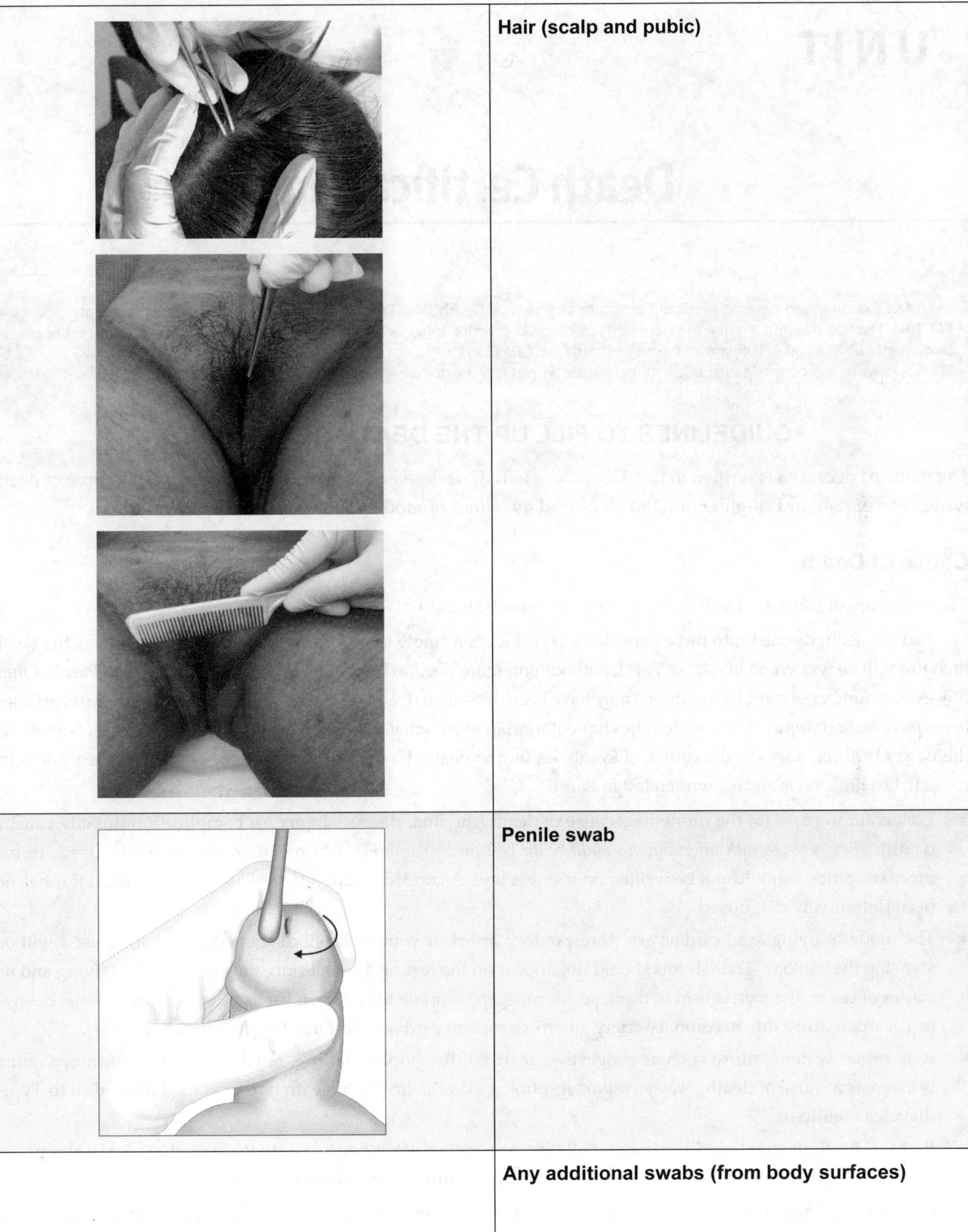

Hair (scalp and pubic)
Penile swab
Any additional swabs (from body surfaces)

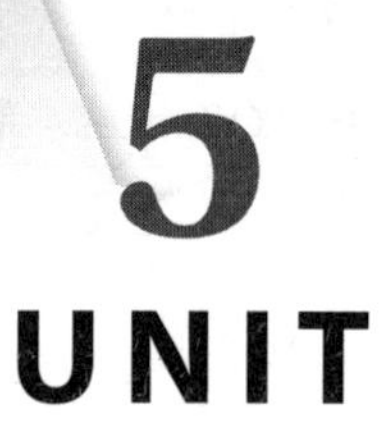

UNIT 5

Death Certification

GUIDELINES TO FILL UP THE DEATH CERTIFICATE

The **name of deceased** is written in full. Do not use initials. If deceased is an infant, not yet named at time of death, write, 'Son of (S/o) or Daughter of (D/o)', followed by names of mother and father.

Cause of Death

The certificate of cause of death is divided into two parts, I and II.

Part I is again divided into three parts, lines (a) (b) (c). If a single morbid condition completely explains the death, then this will be written on line (a) of Part I, and nothing more need to be written in the rest of Part I or in Part II. Often, however, a number of morbid conditions may have been present at death. If so, enter the antecedent causes in Part I, line (b)—the disease or injury that initiated the chain of morbid events that led directly and inevitably to death. Sometimes, there may be three stages in the course of events leading to death. If so, line (c) should be completed. The underlying cause to be tabulated is always written last in Part I.

- First enter in Part I (a) the immediate cause of death (the final disease, injury, or complication directly causing death). *The cause-of-death information should be the best medical opinion.* Abbreviation should not be used. Two or more conditions should not be written on a single line. A condition can be listed as 'probable' even if it has not been definitively diagnosed.

- The mode of dying, e.g., cardiac arrest, respiratory arrest or ventricular fibrillation should not be used without showing the etiology. These terms should not appear on the certificate at all since they are modes of dying and not causes of death. If a mechanism of death seems most appropriate for (a), then list its cause(s) on the line(s) below it (e.g., cardiac arrest **due to** coronary artery atherosclerosis or cardiac arrest **due to** blunt impact to chest).

- If an organ system failure such as congestive heart failure, hepatic failure, renal failure or respiratory failure is listed as a cause of death, always report its etiology on the line(s) beneath it (e.g., renal failure **due to** Type I diabetes mellitus).

Part II *(Other significant conditions):* Enter all diseases or conditions contributing to death that were not reported in the chain of events in Part I and that did not result in the **underlying cause of death**.

Onset: For each cause, indicate the best estimate of the interval between the presumed onset and the date of death. The terms 'unknown' or 'approximately' (e.g., 'from birth', 'several years') may be used. General terms, such as minutes, hours or days are acceptable, if necessary.

Maternal deaths: This information is needed for all women of child-bearing age, even though the pregnancy may have had nothing to do with the death.

Old age or senility: Old age (or senility) should be not given as a cause of death if a more specific cause is known. If old age was contributory factor, it should be entered in Part II.

Manner of Death

Always mention the manner of death since it is important:

a. In determining accurate causes of death
b. In processing insurance claims
c. In statistical studies of injuries and death.

Indicate 'could not be determined' **ONLY** when it is impossible to determine the manner of death.

The following conditions and types of death might seem to be specific or natural but when the medical history is examined further may be found to be complications of an injury or poisoning (possibly occurring long ago). Such cases should be reported to the police.

Epidural/Subarachnoid/Subdural hematoma	Thermal burns/Chemical burns	Open reduction of fracture
Exsanguination	Choking	Drug or alcohol overdose
Fall	Fracture/Hip fracture	Asphyxia
Pulmonary emboli	Hyper-/Hypothermia	Surgery
Seizure disorder	Bolus	Sepsis

MEDICAL CERTIFICATE OF CAUSE OF DEATH

Mr Bachchan Pandey, a 72-year-old male was admitted to the hospital with complaints of severe pain for 1 hour. He had a history of arteriosclerotic heart disease for 8 years with ECG findings of myocardial ischemia and few episodes of congestive cardiac failure. He was on digoxin and diuretics. After admission, blood showed an elevated level of troponin and the ECG showed an acute anterior wall myocardial infarction (MI). Six months before this admission, he was investigated for anemia and occult blood in stool which revealed a large polypoid mass in cecum and diagnosed as carcinoma by biopsy. He was treated with radiation therapy and packed red cell transfusions because of his cardiac status (unfit for surgery). This course was completed 4 months prior to this admission. Treatment for MI started immediately but he expired 1 day later. Fill up the death certificate in this case.

Name of Hospital _____________________________ XXXXXXXX _____________________________

I hereby certify that the person whose particulars are given below died in the hospital ward No. ___ABC___

_____________________________ on _______ 28/02/2024 _______ at _______ 10.30 _______ AM/~~PM~~.

NAME OF DECEASED _____________________ Mr Bachchan Pandey _____________________

Sex	Age at Death			
1. Male ✓ 2. Female	If 1 year or more, age in years 72 years	If less than 1 year, age in months	If less than 1 month, age in days	If less than 1 day, age in hours
		Cause of death		Interval between onset and death (approx)
I. Immediate cause (State the disease, injury or complication, which caused death, not the mode of dying such as heart failure, asthenia, etc.)		Due to (or as a consequences of) a. Acute myocardial infarction		1 day
Antecedent cause (Morbid conditions, if any giving rise to the above cause, stating underlying conditions last)		Due to (or as a consequences of) b. Arteriosclerotic heart disease c. d.		8 years

II. Other significant conditions contributing to the death but not related to the diseases or conditions causing it. Carcinoma cecum, Congestive cardiac failure

Manner of Death: How did the injury occur?
1. Natural ✓   2. Accident   3. Suicide   4. Homicide   5. Pending investigation

If deceased was a female, was pregnancy the death associated with:	1. Yes	2. No ✓
If yes, was there a delivery?	1. Yes	2. No

(Dr Amit Kumar)

Name and signature of the Medical Officer certifying the cause of death ___ PMC No. 12345 ___

Date of verification _______ 28/02/2024 _______

Explanation: Acute MI is listed in Part I (a) as the "Immediate cause of death" which is a direct consequence of "Arteriosclerotic heart disease"—the "Antecedent cause" listed in Part I (b). Carcinoma cecum is listed in Part II as it caused anemia and weakened the patient but it did not cause arteriosclerotic heart disease. Congestive cardiac failure is listed in Part II since it also weakened the heart but it was caused by the atherosclerotic heart disease—it was not part of the sequence leading to acute MI.

EX. 5.1: MEDICAL CERTIFICATE OF CAUSE OF DEATH
(For hospital in-patients, not to be used for stillbirths)

Mrs Ramvati, a 70-year-old obese female was admitted in the ICU with dyspnea and moderate retrosternal pain of 3 hours duration, which did not respond to nitroglycerin. There was a past history of noninsulin-dependent diabetes mellitus, hypertension and episodes of nonexertional chest pain, diagnosed as angina pectoris for 8 years. Over the next 72 hours, she developed a significant elevation of the MB isoenzyme of creatine phosphokinase, confirming an acute myocardial infarction. A Type II second-degree AV block developed, and a temporary pacemaker was put in place. She subsequently developed dyspnea with fluid retention and cardiomegaly on chest radiograph. On the 7th hospital day, during ambulation, she suddenly developed chest pain and increased dyspnea. An acute pulmonary embolism was suspected and intravenous heparin was started. The diagnosis of pulmonary embolism was confirmed by a ventilation/perfusion scan as well as arterial blood gas measurements. One hour later, she became unresponsive and resuscitation efforts were unsuccessful. Fill up the death certificate in this case.

Name of Hospital ____

I hereby certify that the person whose particulars are given below died in the hospital ward No. ___________

___________________________________ on ___________________________ at ___________________ AM/PM.

NAME OF DECEASED ____

Sex	Age at Death			
1. Male 2. Female	If 1 year or more, age in years	If less than 1 year, age in months	If less than 1 month, age in days	If less than 1 day, age in hours
		Cause of death		Interval between onset and death (approx)
I. Immediate cause (State the disease, injury or complication, which caused death, not the mode of dying such as heart failure, asthenia, etc.)		Due to (or as a consequences of) a.		
Antecedent cause (Morbid conditions, if any giving rise to the above cause, stating underlying conditions last)		Due to (or as a consequences of) b. c. d.		
II. Other significant conditions contributing to the death but not related to the diseases or conditions causing it.				
Manner of Death: How did the injury occur? 1. Natural 2. Accident 3. Suicide 4. Homicide 5. Pending investigation				
If deceased was a female, was pregnancy the death associated with: 1. Yes 2. No If yes, was there a delivery? 1. Yes 2. No				

Name and signature of the Medical Officer certifying the cause of death _______________________

Date of verification _______________________

EX. 5.2: MEDICAL CERTIFICATE OF CAUSE OF DEATH
(For hospital in-patients, not to be used for stillbirths)

Ritu Kumari, a 35-year-old gravida three, para two woman with gestational hypertension, reported to the emergency room at 36 weeks into her pregnancy. She had experienced 12 hours of abdominal cramping and vaginal bleeding with the passage of large clots. A presumptive diagnosis of abruptio placenta was made. She continued to bleed from her vagina as well as from phlebotomy sites, and she rapidly went into profound shock. No fetal heart sounds were audible. The patient was experiencing disseminated intravascular coagulation. Despite administration of blood and clotting factors, blood pressure could not be maintained. The mother and fetus both died 1 hour after admission. Fill up the death certificate in this case.

Name of Hospital ____

I hereby certify that the person whose particulars are given below died in the hospital ward No. ___________

_________________________________ on _______________________________ at ___________________ AM/PM.

NAME OF DECEASED ____

Sex	Age at Death			
1. Male 2. Female	If 1 year or more, age in years	If less than 1 year, age in months	If less than 1 month, age in days	If less than 1 day, age in hours
		Cause of death		Interval between onset and death (approx)
I. Immediate cause (State the disease, injury or complication, which caused death, not the mode of dying such as heart failure, asthenia, etc.)		Due to (or as a consequences of) a.		
Antecedent cause (Morbid conditions, if any giving rise to the above cause, stating underlying conditions last)		Due to (or as a consequences of) b. c. d.		

II. Other significant conditions contributing to the death but not related to the diseases or conditions causing it.

Manner of Death: How did the injury occur?
1. Natural   2. Accident   3. Suicide   4. Homicide   5. Pending investigation

If deceased was a female, was pregnancy the death associated with: 1. Yes   2. No
If yes, was there a delivery?   1. Yes   2. No

Name and signature of the Medical Officer certifying the cause of death _____________________________

Date of verification _______________________

EX. 5.3: MEDICAL CERTIFICATE OF CAUSE OF DEATH
(For hospital in-patients, not to be used for stillbirths)

Suresh Prasad, a 65-year-old man slipped and fell down from stairs resulting in fracture of pelvis. After being admitted in hospital, fractures of the left ischium and ilium were reduced. He subsequently developed azotemia, and diagnosed with arteriosclerotic heart disease and pulmonary emphysema. He developed bronchopneumonia after 1 month of his admission and died 5 days later. Autopsy revealed fracture hip and pelvis, cardiac hypertrophy, chronic fibrous myocarditis and coronary atherosclerosis. Prepare a death certificate in this case.

Name of Hospital ____

I hereby certify that the person whose particulars are given below died in the hospital ward No. ___________

_______________________________ on _______________________________ at _____________________ AM/PM.

NAME OF DECEASED ____

Sex	Age at Death			
1. Male 2. Female	If 1 year or more, age in years	If less than 1 year, age in months	If less than 1 month, age in days	If less than 1 day, age in hours
		Cause of death		Interval between onset and death (approx)
I. Immediate cause (State the disease, injury or complication, which caused death, not the mode of dying such as heart failure, asthenia, etc.)	Due to (or as a consequences of) a.			
Antecedent cause (Morbid conditions, if any giving rise to the above cause, stating underlying conditions last)	Due to (or as a consequences of) b. c. d.			
II. Other significant conditions contributing to the death but not related to the diseases or conditions causing it.				
Manner of Death: How did the injury occur? 1. Natural　　2. Accident　　3. Suicide　　4. Homicide　　5. Pending investigation				
If deceased was a female, was pregnancy the death associated with:　　1. Yes　　2. No If yes, was there a delivery?　　1. Yes　　2. No				

Name and signature of the Medical Officer certifying the cause of death _______________________

Date of verification _______________________

EX. 5.4: MEDICAL CERTIFICATE OF CAUSE OF DEATH
(For hospital in-patients, not to be used for stillbirths)

Rony Thomas, a 58-year-old male was admitted in the hospital as his X-ray showed an unusual shadow to the left of sacrum. Further investigations were carried upon. He was diagnosed with adenocarcinoma of the rectum. Further examination and investigations revealed, invasion of the urinary bladder with metastases throughout the abdomen, along with syphilis and decubitus ulcers. Bronchopneumonia developed and the patient died 3 days later. Prepare a death certificate in this case.

Name of Hospital ____

I hereby certify that the person whose particulars are given below died in the hospital ward No. ____________

_________________________________ on _________________________________ at _________________________ AM/PM.

NAME OF DECEASED ____

Sex	Age at Death			
1. Male 2. Female	If 1 year or more, age in years	If less than 1 year, age in months	If less than 1 month, age in days	If less than 1 day, age in hours
		Cause of death		Interval between onset and death (approx)
I. Immediate cause (State the disease, injury or complication, which caused death, not the mode of dying such as heart failure, asthenia, etc.)		Due to (or as a consequences of) a.		
Antecedent cause (Morbid conditions, if any giving rise to the above cause, stating underlying conditions last)		Due to (or as a consequences of) b. c. d.		

II. Other significant conditions contributing to the death but not related to the diseases or conditions causing it.

Manner of Death: How did the injury occur?				
1. Natural	2. Accident	3. Suicide	4. Homicide	5. Pending investigation
If deceased was a female, was pregnancy the death associated with:			1. Yes	2. No
If yes, was there a delivery?			1. Yes	2. No

Name and signature of the Medical Officer certifying the cause of death ___________________________

Date of verification _______________________________

EX. 5.5: MEDICAL CERTIFICATE OF CAUSE OF DEATH
(For hospital in-patients, not to be used for stillbirths)

Vimmi Devi, a 77-year-old female with a 10-year history of hypertension and chronic obstructive pulmonary disease (COPD) presented to the emergency department with complaints of fever, cough and increasing shortness of breath for last 4 days. She reported recent exposure to neighbor with flu-like symptoms, and her wheezing was not improving with her usual bronchodilator therapy. Upon examination, she was febrile, hypoxic, and in moderate respiratory distress. Her chest X-ray demonstrated hyperinflation, and arterial blood gas was consistent with severe respiratory acidosis. Testing of nasal swabs indicated COVID-19. She was admitted to ICU and despite aggressive treatment developed worsening respiratory acidosis and sustained a cardiac arrest on day 3 of admission. Fill up the death certificate in this case.

Name of Hospital ____

I hereby certify that the person whose particulars are given below died in the hospital ward No. _____________

_________________________________ on _________________________________ at _________________________ AM/PM.

NAME OF DECEASED ____

Sex	Age at Death			
1. Male 2. Female	If 1 year or more, age in years	If less than 1 year, age in months	If less than 1 month, age in days	If less than 1 day, age in hours
	Cause of death			Interval between onset and death (approx)
I. Immediate cause (State the disease, injury or complication, which caused death, not the mode of dying such as heart failure, asthenia, etc.)	Due to (or as a consequences of) a.			
Antecedent cause (Morbid conditions, if any giving rise to the above cause, stating underlying conditions last)	Due to (or as a consequences of) b. c. d.			

II. Other significant conditions contributing to the death but not related to the diseases or conditions causing it.

Manner of Death: How did the injury occur?				
1. Natural	2. Accident	3. Suicide	4. Homicide	5. Pending investigation

If deceased was a female, was pregnancy the death associated with:	1. Yes	2. No
If yes, was there a delivery?	1. Yes	2. No

Name and signature of the Medical Officer certifying the cause of death ___________________________

Date of verification _______________________________

EX. 5.6: MEDICAL CERTIFICATE OF CAUSE OF DEATH
(For hospital in-patients, not to be used for stillbirths)

Balwinder, a 45-year-old male had a history of alcohol abuse for 15 years and alcohol induced cirrhosis for about 6 years. He developed portal hypertension 5 months back and he was admitted to the hospital for upper gastrointestinal hemorrhage 3 days back, which endoscopy proved to be due to esophageal varices. Hemorrhage could not be controlled, and he developed shock and cardiac arrest and died. Fill up the death certificate in this case.

Name of Hospital ____

I hereby certify that the person whose particulars are given below died in the hospital ward No. __________

__________________________________ on ____________________________ at ____________________ AM/PM.

NAME OF DECEASED ____

Sex	Age at Death			
1. Male 2. Female	If 1 year or more, age in years	If less than 1 year, age in months	If less than 1 month, age in days	If less than 1 day, age in hours

	Cause of death	Interval between onset and death (approx)
I. Immediate cause (State the disease, injury or complication, which caused death, not the mode of dying such as heart failure, asthenia, etc.)	Due to (or as a consequences of) a.	
Antecedent cause (Morbid conditions, if any giving rise to the above cause, stating underlying conditions last)	Due to (or as a consequences of) b. c. d.	

II. Other significant conditions contributing to the death but not related to the diseases or conditions causing it.

Manner of Death: How did the injury occur?
1. Natural   2. Accident   3. Suicide   4. Homicide   5. Pending investigation

If deceased was a female, was pregnancy the death associated with:	1. Yes	2. No
If yes, was there a delivery?	1. Yes	2. No

Name and signature of the Medical Officer certifying the cause of death ____________________

Date of verification ____________________

6
UNIT

Postmortem Examination

GUIDELINES FOR WRITING AN AUTOPSY REPORT

Autopsy reports: These are medico-legal documents that not only report the anatomic findings of the postmortem examination but which also provide detailed clinic-pathologic correlations. It is important that the autopsy report should contain all the information necessary to support the cause of death statement.

Historical summary: It should include findings in scene investigations, history of incident, medical history, sign and symptoms before death, medical intervention, laboratory findings and imaging findings.

Identification features: Identifying marks and scars (including detailed descriptions of tattoos and healed surgical incisions), body weight and length, hair color and dentition are commonly recorded in unidentified bodies. Fingerprints are taken on separate sheet and attached with the report.

Presentation, clothing, personal effects and associated items: The documentation of how the body was received and the state of the remains before the examination is highly important. The clothing, jewelry and personal effects are to be documented (and photographed). Important areas be encircled on the clothing wherever possible and handed over to the police.

Evidence of medical intervention: All medical devices that were placed in the course of medical therapy should be documented. All tubes, catheters, puncture sites, bandages and other appliances that were placed in the patient are important and places iatrogenic artifacts into context.

Postmortem changes: Documentation of routine postmortem changes aids in interpretation of other autopsy findings. Rigor mortis, algor mortis, postmortem staining and decomposition changes, etc., helps in establishing the postmortem interval and in interpretation of autopsy findings.

External examination: It requires detailed observations organized in a logical manner. Depending on the nature of the case, relevant negatives can be included throughout the report. Descriptions of body height, weight, nutrition, body symmetry, eyes, nose, ears, mouth, teeth, neck, chest, abdomen, genitalia, and extremities give the reader of the report a sense of the condition of the body at the time of the examination, and the quality of the detail gives credence to the overall accuracy and thoroughness of the report.

Internal examination: The internal examination is the central portion of the examination and deserves thoroughness and attention to detail that justifies the autopsy and the original goals of the examination. All internal organs should be inspected, weighed and described. All positive findings should have qualifiers [measurements, color or degree (e.g., mild, moderate, severe)] to give the reader a sense of the magnitude of the abnormality. If there is no disease or injury in the organ examined, it should be mentioned as *'healthy'*. Significant negatives should also be listed based on the peculiarities of the case. General protocol to follow is given in table.

Protocol followed in internal examination

Body cavities (pleural, abdominal, pelvic)	• Organ arrangement • Presence or absence of fluids (straw/turbid/purulent/hemorrhagic), effusions (large/moderate/small) and adhesions (dense/scattered) • Appearance of viscera (degree of decomposition)
Head	• Configuration • Scalp and skull • Weight of brain • Meninges • Hemorrhage, herniations, infection • Blood vessels • Ventricular system • Orbital, nasal and aural cavities • Pituitary
Neck	• General appearance • Mouth, tongue and pharynx • Larynx and vocal cords • Subcutaneous tissue and muscles • Thyroid cartilage • Hyoid bone • Trachea
Respiratory system	• Lung weights • General appearance • Tracheobronchial tree • Parenchyma appearance, with details of diffuse or focal lesions • Diaphragm
Heart	• Weight • Coronary arteries • Valves (including circumferences, if abnormal) • Myocardium (including left and right ventricular wall thickness) • Hemopericardium (quantity) • Aorta and vena cava
GIT	• Esophagus • Stomach (wall condition, contents, quantity and smell) • Pancreas • Small and large intestine (perforation—site, obstruction—cause) • Rectum
Liver and biliary system	• Weight • Color • Consistency • Gallbladder and contents
Reticuloendothelial system	• Spleen weight • Appearance of lymph nodes • Thymus (if present)
Genitourinary tract	• Kidneys (weight and appearance) • Ureters • Bladder and urethra • Male/female genital organs—contusion, abrasion in and around genital organs; in case of male—testes, and in case of female—condition of vagina and ovary, presence of foreign body in uterus, size, products of conception, semen or any other fluid
Musculoskeletal system	• General appearance of all bones, musculature and soft tissues

Histology and microscopic examination: Any tissue may be submitted for examination depending on the nature of the case.

Toxicology, laboratory, and ancillary procedure: The necessary tests should be done since such testing provides important information that is highly important to the final opinion of the cause of death.

POSTMORTEM REPORT

Department of Forensic Medicine and Toxicology
DMC and H, Ludhiana

P.M. Report No. ___DMCH/07–24___   C.R. No. ___________
(in case of hospital admission)

Date and time of receipt of body ___20-03-2024 at 2.30 AM___

Date and time of receipt of inquest papers ___21-03-2024 at 10.30 AM___

Date and time of commencement of autopsy ___21-03-2024 at 11.30 AM___

Time of completion of autopsy ___12.30___ PM

In case of hospital deaths (particular as per hospital records)

Date and time of admission ___________ Date and time of death ___________

Body brought by (Name, signature and rank/number of police official) ___Mahesh Singh___
___Head Constable PC 2284___ Police Station ___Sarabha Nagar, Ludhiana___

Identified by (Name and addresses of relatives/persons acquainted along with their signature)

1. Karnail Singh S/o Rajinder Singh (Father), Vill.: Pakhuwal, Ludhiana
2. Ratan Singh S/o Karnail Singh (Brother), Vill.: Pakhuwal, Ludhiana

History (all events prior to death) As per the information furnished by police, on 20-03-2024 at around 7 pm, the deceased had an argument with his brother over some property matter during dinner time. He was agitated and went to his room and bolted his door. He was found hanging in his room by his wife at 10 pm. He was rushed to DMCH hospital for treatment, but was declared brought dead. [Body was kept in cold storage until commencement of Postmortem examination]

Information furnished by: ___Police___

Particulars of Deceased

Name ___Ranjit singh___ Father's/Husband's Name ___Karnail Singh___

Sex ___M___ Age ___40 years___ Race/Religion ___Sikh___

Address ___Vill.: Pakhuwal, Ludhiana___

Identifications marks (if body is unidentified)

1. Scar mark 1.2 cm × 0.1 cm placed obliquely over anterior surface of left forearm, 8" below elbow joint and 9.2" above wrist joint.
2. Black mole of 0.2 cm × 0.1 cm size placed over right side ala of nose, 1.1 cm behind the tip of the nose.

Height ___178___ cm   Weight ___80___ kg

Circumcision: Yes/No   Beard, mustache ___No___

____
Signature of the Doctor

SCHEDULE OF OBSERVATIONS

A. General	
Body	Entire and intact/Mutilated and in pieces
Clothings	Pant, underwear, shirt and vest. Front of shirt showing dried marks of dribbling of saliva on right side
Medical intervention (if any)	Hospital injection marks present over the right cubital fossa and right dorsum of hand
Built	Well/Moderate/Poor/Emaciated
Nourishment/Physique	Lean/Medium/Obese
Scars/Tattoos/Bedsores (if present)	NIL
Skin	Pallor/Jaundiced/Pink/Cyanosis/Normal (Cyanosis of palms)
Facial appearance	Pale/Normal/Livid/Cyanosed

Eyes
   Cornea
   Pupils
   Conjunctivae
	Closed/Half open/Open
	Clear/Hazy/Opaque Arcus senilis: Absent/Developing/Fully developed
	Constricted/Dilated Regular/Irregular
	Pale/Normal/Congested/Jaundiced/Hemorrhagic
	Subconjunctival hemorrhages seen

Nostrils	Bloodstained froth
Ears	Cyanosed earlobes
Mouth	Slightly open, dried marks of saliva present from right angle of mouth
Teeth	Clenched
Tongue	Protruding and caught in between teeth
Oral cavity	NAD

Circum-oral regions
   Lips
   Inner aspects of lips
   Frenulum
	
	Pale/Cyanosed
	NAD
	Cyanosed/Torn/NAD

Orifice
   Urethral
   Anal
   Vaginal (in females)
	
	Dried seminal discharge present on external urethral meatus and prepare
	NAD

Condition of limbs	Cyanosis of palms of hands and nail beds
Rigor mortis	Developing/Fully developed/Passing off Mild/Strong
Postmortem staining	Fixed/Not fixed Areas present <u>Both forearms, lower limbs and back (faint)</u>

Decomposition changes
   Skin
   Face/Abdomen/Scrotum
   Foul smell
   Maggots
	Absent
	Color changes of putrefaction/Marbling/Skin slippage/NAD
	Bloated/Not bloated
	Present/Absent
	Present/Absent

Any other findings	

____

Signature of the Doctor

B. External Injuries*

(Mention type, shape, length × breadth × depth of each injury and its relation to important body landmark. Indicate which injuries are fresh and which are old and their duration)

Ligature mark is present obliquely above the thyroid cartilage over the front and sides of the neck and extending towards the back of the neck in an upward and backward direction with sparing of the left side neck in the form of inverted "V" near the angle of mandible. The ligature mark is 34 × 2 cm in size, and is located 5 cm below the chin, 4 cm below the left ear lobe, 7 cm below the right ear lobe and is discontinuous on the back of the neck for 8 cm (the same is depicted in pictograph as "1").

Ligature mark is yellowish brown in color, dry and parchmentized with multiple reddish abrasions on its upper border. The neck is tilted towards the right side with apparent lengthening of the neck. The skin around the ligature mark is showing redness.

On dissection, there is glistening white band underneath the ligature mark with fracture of greater cornu of hyoid on the right side. There is hemorrhage around the fracture site. Carotid artery on the left side shows intimal tear.

The strap muscles of the neck and thyroid cartilage are intact. No other injuries or marks of restraint are present.

(Ligature material is not there in situ or brought to the postmortem examination center).

C. Internal Examination

Head	
Scalp	Petechial hemorrhages all over the scalp
Skull	NAD (No abnormality detected)
Brain	1500 gm, congested. Cut section showed petechial hemorrhages in the white matter
Neck	As described above
Chest	
Ribs/Sternum/Chest wall	Intact, NAD
Pleura and Pleural cavities	Adherent to chest wall on right side
Trachea and Larynx	Congested, intact
Lungs	
Right	Congested and edematous, 650 gm ⎤ Cut section exuded frothy blood
Left	Congested and edematous, 600 gm ⎦
Pericardium	No organic changes. No evidence of petechiae or any organic changes
Heart	Congested, contains dark colored fluid blood
Coronaries	Patent, NAD
Large blood vessels	Contains dark colored fluid blood
Abdomen	
Peritoneum	Normal, intact
Stomach and its contents	Contains undigested rice and potatoes. Smell is unremarkable, mucosa NAD
Small intestines and its contents	Empty, mucosa congested
Large intestines and its contents	Contains fecal matter and gas, mucosa slightly congested
Liver	1550 gm, congested, intact
Gallbladder	Distended
Spleen	160 gm, congested, intact
Pancreas	Intact, NAD
Kidneys and ureters	R: 130 gm ⎤ Intact and congested
	L: 130 gm ⎦
Urinary bladder	Empty, NAD
Pelvic cavity	Intact, NAD

____

Signature of the Doctor

____

* Injuries are to be given in serial number and mark them on the diagrams attached. In stab injuries, mention angles, margins and direction inside the body. In firearms injuries, mention direction and effects of fire.

Genital organs	Intact, NAD
Spinal columns and spinal cord (opened where indicated)	NAD

OPINION

a. Probable time since death (keeping all factors including observations at inquest)

  i. Between injury and death ________________ Within few minutes ________________

  ii. Between death and postmortem examination ________ 12 to 24 hours ________

b. Cause and manner of death. The cause of death to the best of my knowledge and belief is:

  i. Immediate cause ________________ Asphyxia ________________

  ii. Due to ________________ Antemortem hanging ________________

  iii. Which of the injuries are antemortem/postmortem and duration if antemortem? Antemortem ________

  ____

  iv. Manner of causation of injuries (if possible) ____________ Suicidal ________

  v. Whether injuries (individually or collectively) are sufficient to cause death in ordinary course of nature or

  not? Injury is sufficient to cause death in ordinary course of nature ________

c. Any other ____

Specimens collected and preserved* *(Tick '✓')*

☐ Viscera (1. Stomach and small intestines with its contents, 2. Part of liver, half of each kidneys 3. Blood 4. Urine 5. Preservative used for sample 1 and 2, 6. Preservative used for sample 3 and 4)
☐ Sample of blood in gauze piece (dried)
☐ Clothes (air dried)
☐ Photographs/Video CD in case of custody deaths/Fingerprints
☐ Foreign body (like bullet, ligature)
☐ Slides from vagina or any other material _______________________________
☐ Organs for histopathological examination

Dr Amit Kumar
PMC No. 12345
____

Place Ludhiana

Signature of the Doctor
Name (block letters), Designation and Seal

____

Received PM report No. ________________________________ in original/copy along with body diagram and

________________________ inquest papers (mention total number and initial them all).

(Viscera or any other specimen, if preserved is handed over to the police immediately after autopsy)

Name ________________________ P.C. No. ________________________ P.S. ________________________

____

Signature and Date

____

* Depending upon the crime scene, history, findings, and autopsy surgeon's observations, the viscera is preserved in suspected case of hanging.

Date _21-03-2024_   **PMR No.** _DMCH/07-24_

Right Side   Front   Back   Left Side

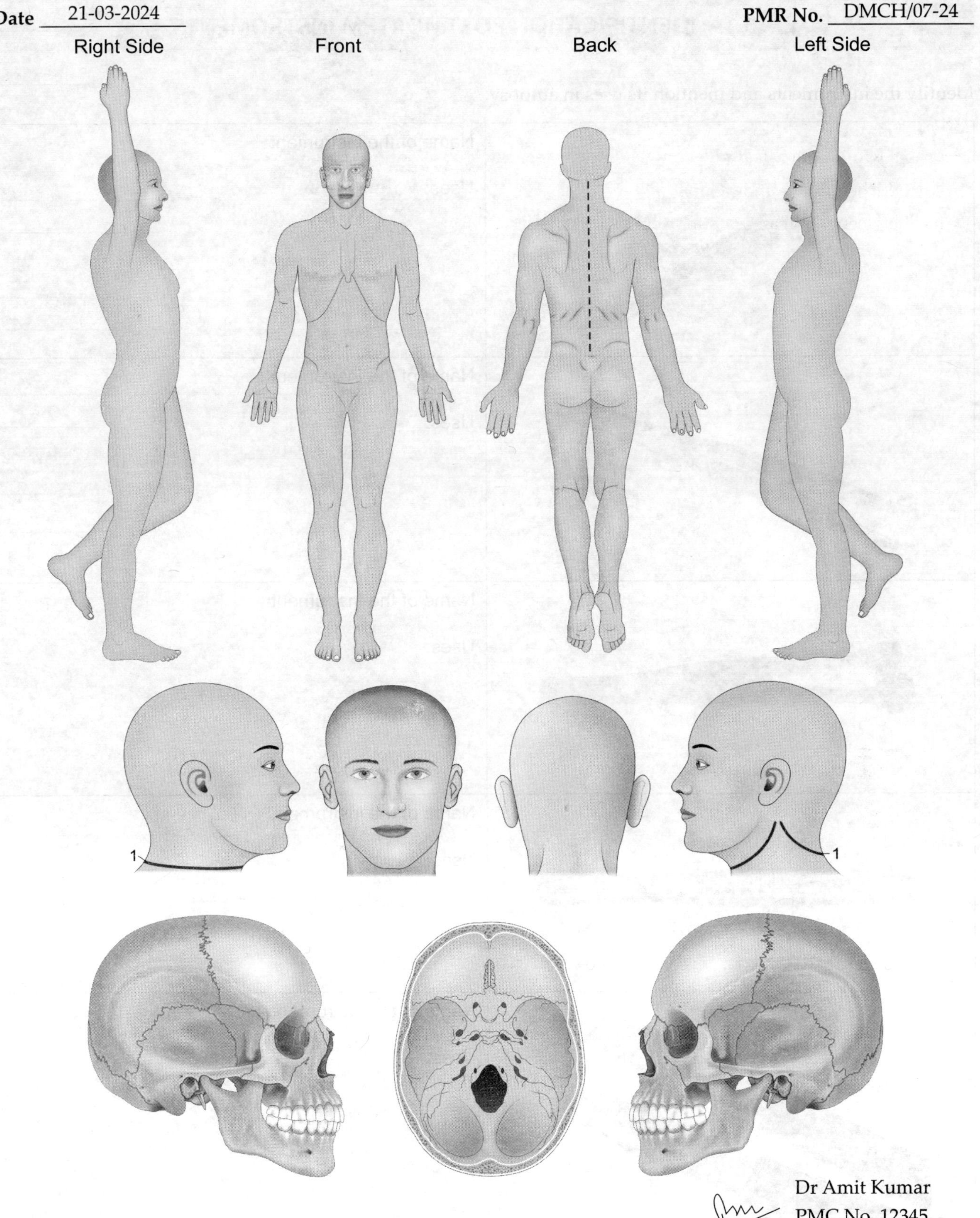

Dr Amit Kumar
PMC No. 12345

Signature of the Doctor
Name, Designation and Seal

EX. 6.1A: IDENTIFICATION POSTMORTEM INSTRUMENTS

Identify the instruments and mention its uses in autopsy.

	Name of the instrument: Uses:
	Name of the instrument: Uses:
	Name of the instrument: Uses:
	Name of the instrument: Uses:
	Name of the instrument: Uses:

EX. 6.1B: IDENTIFICATION POSTMORTEM INSTRUMENTS

Identify the instruments and mention its uses in autopsy.

	Name of the instrument: Uses:
	Name of the instrument: Uses:
	Name of the instrument: Uses:
	Name of the instrument: Uses:

EX. 6.1C: IDENTIFICATION POSTMORTEM INSTRUMENTS

Identify the instruments and mention its uses in autopsy.

	Name of the instrument: Uses:
	Name of the instrument: Uses:
	Name of the instrument: Uses:
	Name of the instrument: Uses:
	Name of the instrument: Uses:

EX. 6.1D: IDENTIFICATION POSTMORTEM INSTRUMENTS

Identify the instruments and mention its uses in autopsy.

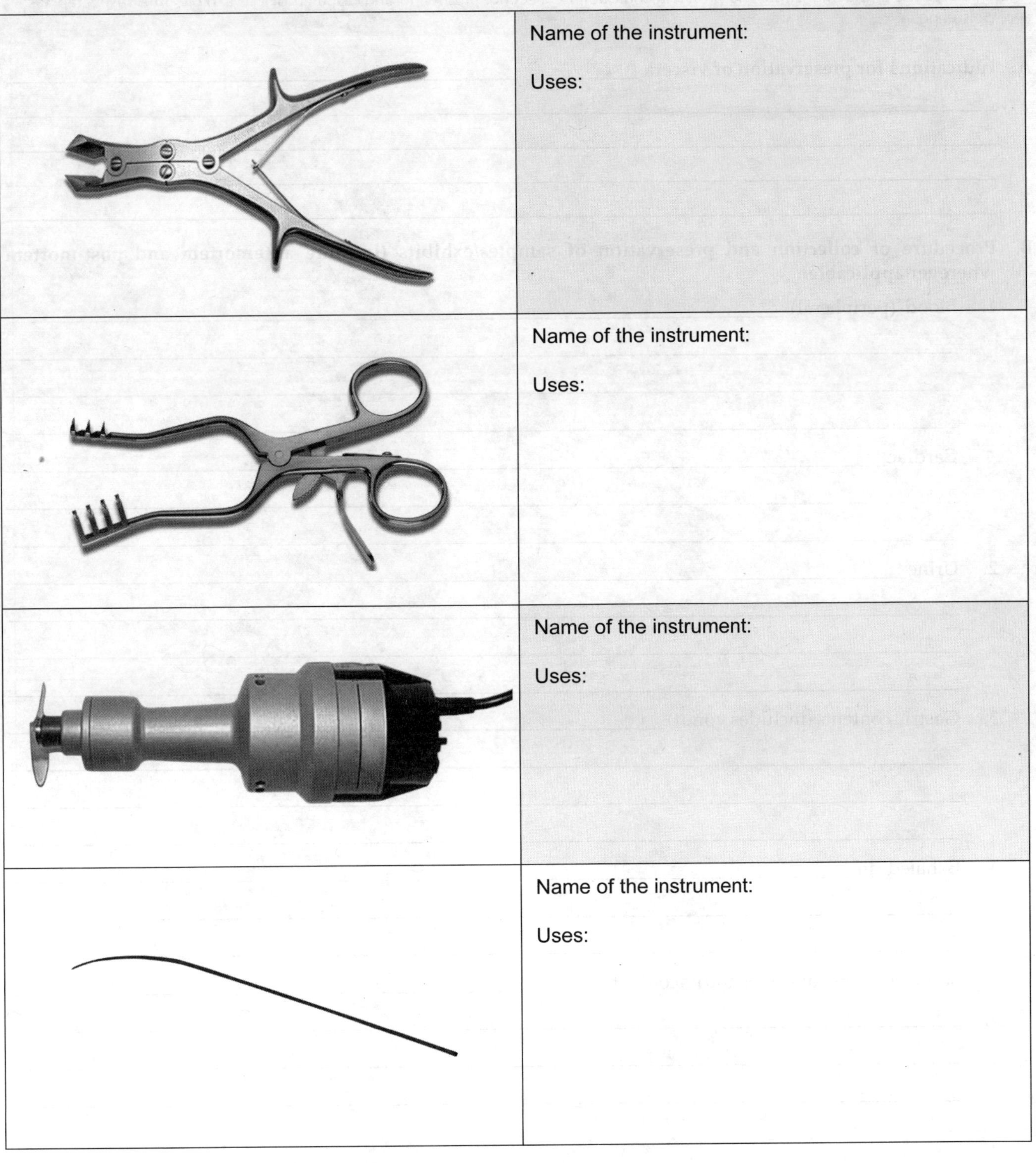

	Name of the instrument: Uses:
	Name of the instrument: Uses:
	Name of the instrument: Uses:
	Name of the instrument: Uses:

EX. 6.2: COLLECTION, PRESERVATION AND DISPATCH OF THE EXHIBITS IN CASE OF POISONING

FM 14.3: Assist and demonstrate the proper technique in collecting, preserving and dispatch of the exhibits in a suspected case of poisoning.

A. Indications for preservation of viscera ____

____

____

____

____

B. Procedure of collection and preservation of samples/exhibits (indicate antemortem and post-mortem wherever applicable):

1. Blood (peripheral) ____

    ____

    ____

    Cardiac____

    ____

    ____

2. Urine____

    ____

    ____

    ____

3. Gastric contents (includes vomit) ____

    ____

    ____

    ____

4. Exhaled air____

    ____

    ____

5. Stomach, small intestines and its contents__________________________________

    ____

    ____

    ____

    ____

6. Liver and gallbladder

7. Kidneys

8. Spleen

9. Cerebrospinal fluid

10. Vitreous humor

11. Brain

12. Lungs

13. Heart

14. Uterus and appendages

15. Skin

16. Maggots____

____

____

17. Skeletal muscle_______________________________________

____

____

18. Bone____

____

____

19. Head hair____

____

____

20. Finger and toe nails___________________________________

____

____

21. Fat____

____

____

22. Saliva____

____

____

23. Others____

____

____

EX. 6.3: POSTMORTEM EXAMINATION OF FETUS

FM 14.12: To estimate the age of fetus by postmortem examination.

A female fetus of 49 cm crown heel length was brought to the mortuary with alleged history of killing of the baby after home delivery. But the mother claims it to be stillborn and is 1 month premature. Write a detailed autopsy report for the same.

Report No. _______________________________   Date _______________

Name _____________________________________ S/D of _____________________________

Address ____

Body identified by ______________________ Police personnel _____________________

Police Station ______________________________ District _______________________

EXTERNAL EXAMINATION

Clothings and wrappings (describe) ____

Length (cm)__________   Weight (gm) ____________   Foot length (cm) ______________

Circumference (cm): Head ________________ Chest _________________ Abdominal ______________

Sex (Male-M/Female-F/Ambiguous-A/Undifferentiated-U) [ ]

Hair	Scalp hair _____________________ Lanugo hair: Present (mention areas) ______________/Absent Eyebrows: Present/Absent Eyelashes: Present/Absent Adherent/Separated
Vernix caseosa	Present (mention areas) ______________/Absent
Skin	Normal/Wrinkled/Macerated/Decomposed Surface injuries ________________ Other (describe) ________
Head	Normal/Hydrocephalic/Scalp defects/Anencephalic/Abnormal skull shape/Collapsed/Molding Trauma ________________________ Other (describe) ____________
Eyes	Normal/Close together/Far apart/Straight/Up slanting/Down slanting/Abnormally small/ Abnormally large/Epicanthus Other (describe) ___________ Conjunctiva ________________
Nose	Normal/Other (describe) ________________________ Injuries ____________________________
Mouth	Normal/Cleft palate/Cleft lip/Large tongue/Small chin Injuries ____________ Other (describe) ___________

Ears	Normal/Lowest/Tags/Pits/Symmetric Level of crest with lateral canthus __________	Plasticity _______________________ Other (describe) ____________
Neck	Normal/Excess skin/Cystic mass Injuries _______________________________	Other (describe) ____________
Chest	Normal/Asymmetric/Small/Other _________	
Abdomen	Normal/Distended/Omphalocele/Gastroschisis/Hernia/3-vessel cord Other ____	
Back	Normal/Spina bifida (defect level ______)/Scoliosis/Kyphosis Other (describe) _______________________________	

Limbs	Length (Normal/Short/Long)	Form (Normal/Symmetric/Missing parts)	Position (Normal/Abnormal)
Arms			
Right			
Left			
Legs			
Right			
Left			

Hands		
Right	Fingers ( ), Webbing/Syndactyly/Transverse crease	Other ____________
Left	Fingers ( ), Webbing/Syndactyly/Transverse crease	Other ____________
Feet		
Right	Toes ( ), Webbing/Wide space between toes 1–2	Other ____________
Left	Toes ( ), Webbing/Wide space between toes 1–2	Other ____________
Nails	Normal/Small (which ones?) _______________ Level with fingers _______________	Other ____________
Genitalia	Normal/Imperforate anus Ambiguous genitalia (describe) ______________________	
Male	Hypospadias/Chordee/Undescended testes (right/left) ________________ Other (describe) _____________	
Female	Normal/Abnormal urethral opening Clitoromegaly: Yes/No Other (describe) ____________	

Injuries (any other/burns/fracture): ____

____

____

____

Any other mass (Yes/No), if yes, describe ____

INTERNAL EXAMINATION

Head and Neck

Scalp:

Cephalhematoma and caput succedaneum:

Fontanelles:

Skull:

Meninges:

Brain:

Neck:

Thorax

Level of diaphragm:

Thymus:

Pleura:

Lungs: Wt (gm) Right __________ Left __________ Volume ______________ Margins ________

    Consistency: Crepitant/Noncrepitant   Color: Reddish brown/Salmon-pink

    Sectioning: Frothless blood/Frothy blood

    Hydrostatic test:

Heart: Wt (gm) ________

    Condition of valves:

    Foramen ovale:

Abdomen

Stomach (contents):

Intestines (meconium presence and site):

Liver: Size (cm) __________ Wt (gm) __________ Consistency: Soft/Firm/Hard

Gallbladder: Absent/Present

Spleen: Size (cm) __________ Wt (gm) __________ Consistency: Soft/Firm/Hard

Kidneys: Size (cm) Right__________ Left __________

         Wt (gm) Right __________ Left __________

Ureters:

Urinary bladder:

OSSIFICATION CENTERS *(Tick '✓')*

☐ Calcaneum   ☐ Sternum   ☐ Talus

☐ Lower end of femur   ☐ Upper end of tibia

UMBILICAL CORD

Umbilical cord length (cm) _____________   Normal/Abnormal

Umbilical vessels _____________________ Condition of cord _____________________

PLACENTA EXAMINATION

Weight (gm) _____________________   Diameter (cm) _____________________

Morphology: Normal/Abnormal

Cord insertion: Normal/Abnormal   Infarct Yes/No

Chorionicity of multiple pregnancy _____________________

Membrane culture   Negative/Positive

Histopathology Done/Not done   Suggestive of syphilis   Yes/No

PRESERVATION OF SAMPLES (for DNA, blood grouping and toxicological screening)

1. ____

2. ____

3. ____

OPINION

____

____

____

____

Place ___________   Signature of the Doctor

Date ___________   Name, Designation and Seal

Received PM report No. _____________________ along with _____________________ number of envelopes and

_____________________ number of samples and sample seal.

Name _____________________ P.C. No. _____________________ P.S. _____________________

____

Signature and Date

EX. 6.3A: FETAL EXAMINATION FOR INTRAUTERINE AGE

FM 14.12: To estimate the age of fetus by postmortem examination.

Age (in months)	Features/Findings

Rule of Hasse ____

____

EX. 6.4.1: POSTMORTEM REPORT

FM 14.6: Conduct and prepare postmortem examination report of varied etiologies (at least 15) in a simulated/supervised environment.

Department of Forensic Medicine and Toxicology

____

P.M. Report No. _______________   C.R. No. ___________________
                                                                               (in case of hospital admission)

Date and time of receipt of body ______________________________

Date and time of receipt of inquest papers ________________

Date and time of commencement of autopsy ___________________

Time of completion of autopsy ___________ AM/PM

In case of hospital deaths (particular as per hospital records)

Date and time of admission _________________ Date and time of death _________________

Body brought by (Name, signature and rank/number of police official) _______________________________

____ Police Station ______________________________

Identified by (Name and addresses of relatives/persons acquainted along with their signature)

1. ____

2. ____

History (all events prior to death) _______________________________________

____

____

Information furnished by: ___________________________________

Particulars of Deceased

Name _________________________________ Father's/Husband's Name _____________________________

Sex _____________________ Age _________________ Race/Religion _______________________

Address ____

Identifications marks (if body is unidentified)

1. ____

2. ____

Height _____________ cm   Weight _____________ kg

Circumcision: Yes/No   Beard, mustache ___________________

____

                                                                   Signature of the Doctor

SCHEDULE OF OBSERVATIONS

A. General	
Body	Entire and intact/Mutilated and in pieces
Clothings	
Medical intervention (if any)	
Built	Well/Moderate/Poor/Emaciated
Nourishment/Physique	Lean/Medium/Obese
Scars/Tattoos/Bedsores (if present)	
Skin	Pallor/Jaundiced/Pink/Cyanosis/Normal
Facial appearance	Pale/Normal/Livid/Cyanosed
Eyes	Closed/Half open/Open
Cornea	Clear/Hazy/Opaque Arcus senilis: Absent/Developing/Fully developed
Pupils	Constricted/Dilated Regular/Irregular
Conjunctivae	Pale/Normal/Congested/Jaundiced/Hemorrhagic
Nostrils	
Ears	
Mouth	
Teeth	
Tongue	
Oral cavity	
Circum-oral regions	
Lips	Pale/Cyanosed
Inner aspects of lips	
Frenulum	Intact/Torn
Orifice	
Urethral	
Anal	
Vaginal (in females)	
Condition of limbs	
Rigor mortis	Developing/Fully developed/Passing off Mild/Strong
Postmortem staining	Fixed/Not fixed Areas present_______________
Decomposition changes	
Skin	Color changes of putrefaction/Marbling/Skin slippage
Face/Abdomen/Scrotum	Bloated/Not bloated
Foul smell	Present/Absent
Maggots	Present/Absent
Any other findings	

Signature of the Doctor

B. External Injuries*
(Mention type, shape, length × breadth × depth of each injury and its relation to important body landmark. Indicate which injuries are fresh and which are old and their duration)

C. Internal Examination	

Head
  Scalp
  Skull
  Brain	

Neck	

Chest
  Ribs/Sternum/Chest wall
  Pleural cavities
  Lungs
    Right
    Left
  Pericardium
  Heart
    Coronaries
    Large blood vessels	

Abdomen
  Peritoneum
 	
  Stomach and its contents
 	
  Small intestines and its contents
 	
  Large intestines and its contents
 	
  Liver
 	
  Gallbladder
  Spleen
 	
  Pancreas
  Kidneys and ureters
 	
  Urinary bladder
  Pelvic cavity	

Signature of the Doctor

---

* Injuries are to be given in serial number and mark them on the diagrams attached. In stab injuries, mention angles, margins and direction inside the body. In firearms injuries, mention direction and effects of fire.

Genital organs	
Spinal columns and spinal cord (opened where indicated)	

OPINION

a. Probable time since death (keeping all factors including observations at inquest)

   i.   Between injury and death ____

   ii. Between death and postmortem examination ____

b. Cause and manner of death. The cause of death to the best of my knowledge and belief is:

   i.   Immediate cause ____

   ii. Due to ____

   iii. Which of the injuries are antemortem/postmortem and duration if antemortem? ____________

       ____

   iv. Manner of causation of injuries (if possible) _______________________________________

   v. Whether injuries (individually or collectively) are sufficient to cause death in ordinary course of nature or not? ____

c. Any other ____

Specimens collected and preserved *(Tick '✓')*

☐ Viscera (1. Stomach and small intestines with its contents, 2. Part of liver, half of each kidneys 3. Blood 4. Urine 5. Preservative used for sample 1 and 2, 6. Preservative used for sample 3 and 4)
☐ Sample of blood in gauze piece (dried)
☐ Clothes (air dried)
☐ Photographs/Video CD in case of custody deaths/Fingerprints
☐ Foreign body (like bullet, ligature)
☐ Slides from vagina or any other material ____
☐ Organs for histopathological examination

Place __________

____
Signature of the Doctor
Name (block letters), Designation and Seal

____

Received PM report No. _______________________________ in original/copy along with body diagram and

_______________________________ inquest papers (mention total number and initial them all).

(Viscera or any other specimen, if preserved is handed over to the police immediately after autopsy)

Name _______________________ P.C. No. _______________________ P.S. _______________

____
Signature and Date

Date _______________

PMR No. _______________

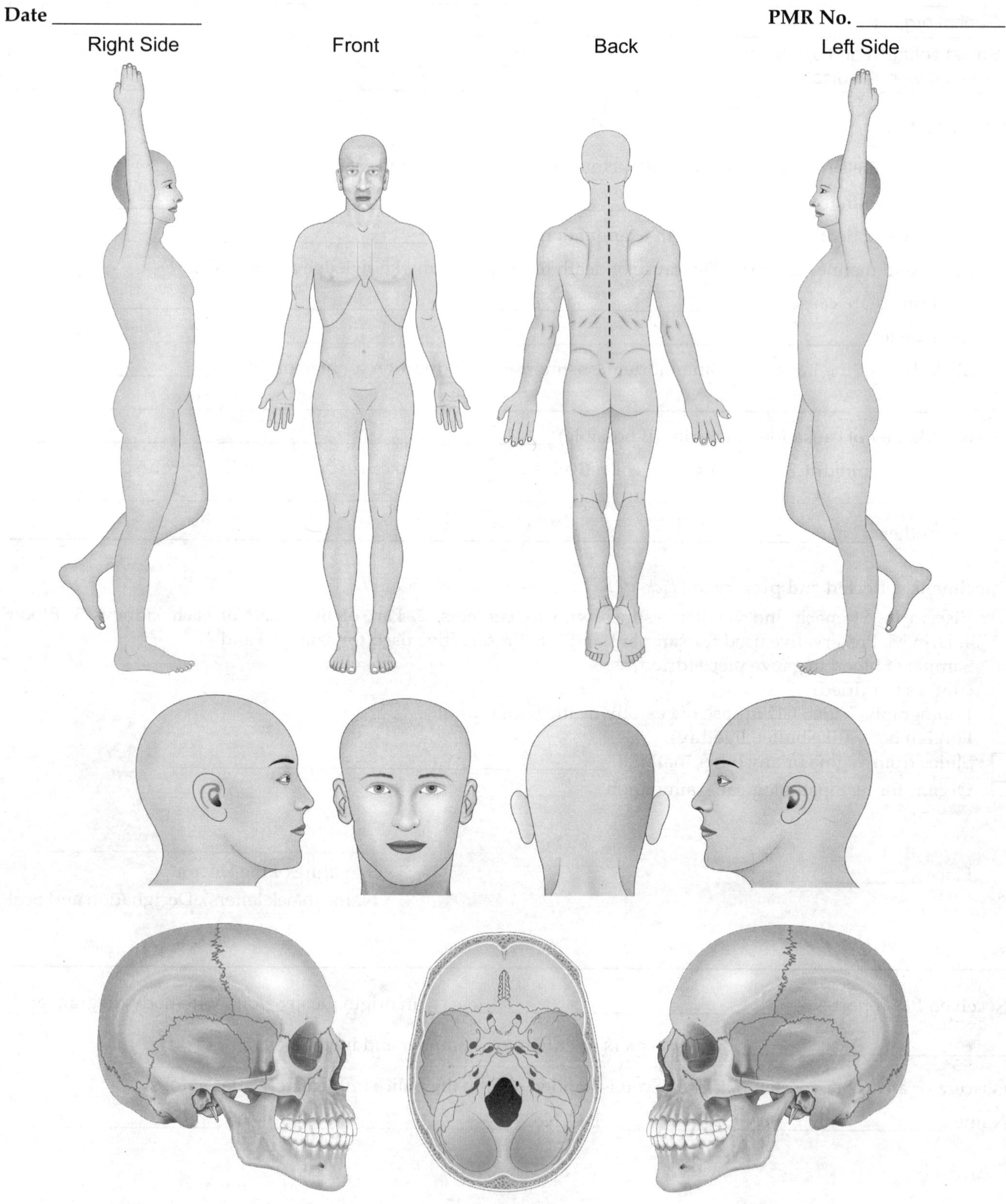

____
Signature of the Doctor
Name, Designation and Seal

EX. 6.4.2: POSTMORTEM REPORT

Department of Forensic Medicine and Toxicology

____

P.M. Report No. _________________   C.R. No. _________________
                                           (in case of hospital admission)

Date and time of receipt of body _____________________

Date and time of receipt of inquest papers _______________

Date and time of commencement of autopsy _________________

Time of completion of autopsy ___________ AM/PM

In case of hospital deaths (particular as per hospital records)

Date and time of admission ________________ Date and time of death _________________

Body brought by (Name, signature and rank/number of police official) _______________________________

____ Police Station ________________________________

Identified by (Name and addresses of relatives/persons acquainted along with their signature)

1. ____

2. ____

History (all events prior to death) ____

____

____

Information furnished by: _______________________________________

Particulars of Deceased

Name _______________________________ Father's/Husband's name _______________________________

Sex _________________________ Age ________________ Race/Religion _______________________________

Address ____

Identifications marks (if body is unidentified)

1. ____

2. ____

Height _______________ cm   Weight _______________ kg

Circumcision: Yes/No   Beard, mustache _________________

____

Signature of the Doctor

SCHEDULE OF OBSERVATIONS

A. General	
Body	Entire and intact/Mutilated and in pieces
Clothings	
Medical intervention (if any)	
Built	Well/Moderate/Poor/Emaciated
Nourishment/Physique	Lean/Medium/Obese
Scars/Tattoos/Bedsores (if present)	
Skin	Pallor/Jaundiced/Pink/Cyanosis/Normal
Facial appearance	Pale/Normal/Livid/Cyanosed

Eyes
  Cornea
  Pupils
  Conjunctivae
	Closed/Half open/Open
	Clear/Hazy/Opaque Arcus senilis: Absent/Developing/Fully developed
	Constricted/Dilated Regular/Irregular
	Pale/Normal/Congested/Jaundiced/Hemorrhagic

Nostrils	
Ears	
Mouth	
Teeth	
Tongue	
Oral cavity	

Circum-oral regions
  Lips
  Inner aspects of lips
  Frenulum
	
	Pale/Cyanosed
	
	Intact/Torn

Orifice
  Urethral
  Anal
  Vaginal (in females)	

Condition of limbs	
Rigor mortis	Developing/Fully developed/Passing off Mild/Strong
Postmortem staining	Fixed/Not fixed Areas present______________

Decomposition changes
  Skin
  Face/Abdomen/Scrotum
  Foul smell
  Maggots
	
	Color changes of putrefaction/Marbling/Skin slippage
	Bloated/Not bloated
	Present/Absent
	Present/Absent

Any other findings	

Signature of the Doctor

B. External Injuries*
(Mention type, shape, length × breadth × depth of each injury and its relation to important body landmark. Indicate which injuries are fresh and which are old and their duration)

C. Internal Examination	

Head
  Scalp
  Skull
  Brain	

Neck	

Chest
  Ribs/Sternum/Chest wall
  Pleural cavities
  Lungs
    Right
    Left
  Pericardium
  Heart
    Coronaries
    Large blood vessels	

Abdomen
  Peritoneum
 	
  Stomach and its contents
 	
  Small intestines and its contents
 	
  Large intestines and its contents
 	
  Liver
 	
  Gallbladder
  Spleen
 	
  Pancreas
  Kidneys and ureters
 	
  Urinary bladder
  Pelvic cavity	

Signature of the Doctor

* Injuries are to be given in serial number and mark them on the diagrams attached. In stab injuries, mention angles, margins and direction inside the body. In firearms injuries, mention direction and effects of fire.

Genital organs	
Spinal columns and spinal cord (opened where indicated)	

OPINION

a.   Probable time since death (keeping all factors including observations at inquest)

   i.   Between injury and death ____

   ii. Between death and postmortem examination ________________________________

b.   Cause and manner of death. The cause of death to the best of my knowledge and belief is:

   i.   Immediate cause ____

   ii. Due to ____

   iii. Which of the injuries are antemortem/postmortem and duration if antemortem? _____________

      ____

   iv. Manner of causation of injuries (if possible) ______________________________________

   v. Whether injuries (individually or collectively) are sufficient to cause death in ordinary course of nature or not? ____

c.   Any other ____

Specimens collected and preserved (*Tick '✓'*)

☐ Viscera (1. Stomach and small intestines with its contents, 2. Part of liver, half of each kidneys 3. Blood 4. Urine 5. Preservative used for sample 1 and 2, 6. Preservative used for sample 3 and 4)
☐ Sample of blood in gauze piece (dried)
☐ Clothes (air dried)
☐ Photographs/Video CD in case of custody deaths/Fingerprints
☐ Foreign body (like bullet, ligature)
☐ Slides from vagina or any other material _______________________________________
☐ Organs for histopathological examination

Place __________

Signature of the Doctor
Name (block letters), Designation and Seal

Received PM report No. ________________________________ in original/copy along with body diagram and

________________________ inquest papers (mention total number and initial them all).

(Viscera or any other specimen, if preserved is handed over to the police immediately after autopsy)

Name ___________________________ P.C. No. ____________________ P.S. ________________

Signature and Date

Date ______________

PMR No. ______________

| Right Side | Front | Back | Left Side |

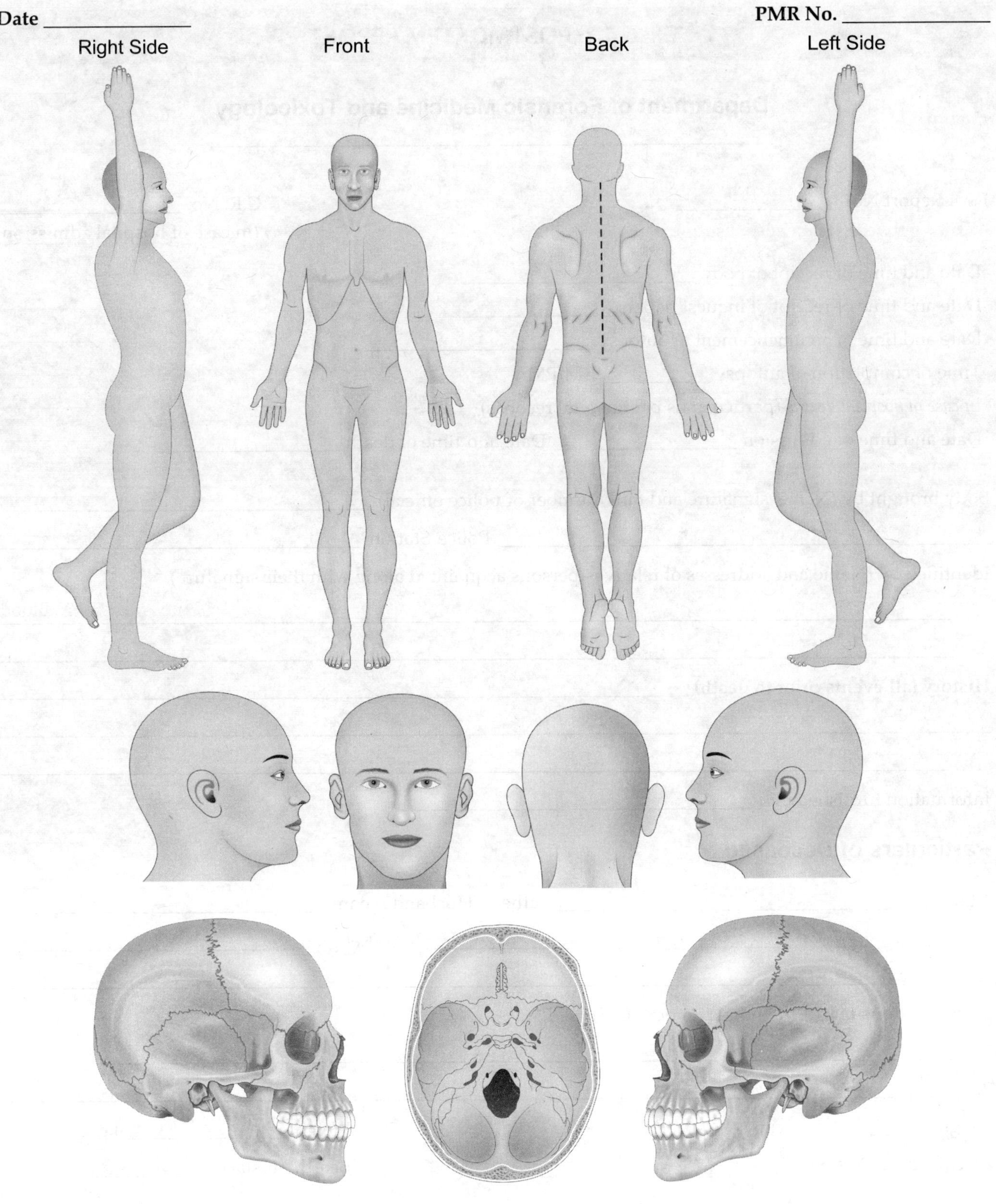

____
Signature of the Doctor
Name, Designation and Seal

EX. 6.4.3: POSTMORTEM REPORT

Department of Forensic Medicine and Toxicology

____

P.M. Report No. _________________   C.R. No. _________________

(in case of hospital admission)

Date and time of receipt of body _____________________

Date and time of receipt of inquest papers _______________

Date and time of commencement of autopsy ___________________

Time of completion of autopsy ___________ AM/PM

In case of hospital deaths (particular as per hospital records)

Date and time of admission _________________ Date and time of death _________________

Body brought by (Name, signature and rank/number of police official) _____________________

_______________________________________ Police Station _____________________________

Identified by (Name and addresses of relatives/persons acquainted along with their signature)

1. ____

2. ____

History (all events prior to death) ____

____

____

Information furnished by: _______________________________

Particulars of Deceased

Name ___________________________ Father's/Husband's name _____________________

Sex ___________________ Age _________________ Race/Religion _____________________

Address ____

Identifications marks (if body is unidentified)

1. ____

2. ____

Height _____________ cm   Weight _____________ kg

Circumcision: Yes/No   Beard, mustache _________________

____
Signature of the Doctor

SCHEDULE OF OBSERVATIONS

A. General	
Body	Entire and intact/Mutilated and in pieces
Clothings	
Medical intervention (if any)	
Built	Well/Moderate/Poor/Emaciated
Nourishment/Physique	Lean/Medium/Obese
Scars/Tattoos/Bedsores (if present)	
Skin	Pallor/Jaundiced/Pink/Cyanosis/Normal
Facial appearance	Pale/Normal/Livid/Cyanosed

Eyes
   Cornea
   Pupils
   Conjunctivae
	Closed/Half open/Open
	Clear/Hazy/Opaque Arcus senilis: Absent/Developing/Fully developed
	Constricted/Dilated Regular/Irregular
	Pale/Normal/Congested/Jaundiced/Hemorrhagic

Nostrils	
Ears	
Mouth	
Teeth	
Tongue	
Oral cavity	

Circum-oral regions
   Lips
   Inner aspects of lips
   Frenulum
	
	Pale/Cyanosed
	
	Intact/Torn

Orifice
   Urethral
   Anal
   Vaginal (in females)	

Condition of limbs	
Rigor mortis	Developing/Fully developed/Passing off Mild/Strong
Postmortem staining	Fixed/Not fixed Areas present__________________

Decomposition changes
   Skin
   Face/Abdomen/Scrotum
   Foul smell
   Maggots
	
	Color changes of putrefaction/Marbling/Skin slippage
	Bloated/Not bloated
	Present/Absent
	Present/Absent

Any other findings	

Signature of the Doctor

B. External Injuries*
(Mention type, shape, length × breadth × depth of each injury and its relation to important body landmark. Indicate which injuries are fresh and which are old and their duration)

C. Internal Examination	

Head
  Scalp
  Skull
  Brain	

Neck	

Chest
  Ribs/Sternum/Chest wall
  Pleural cavities
  Lungs
    Right
    Left
  Pericardium
  Heart
    Coronaries
    Large blood vessels	

Abdomen
  Peritoneum
 	
  Stomach and its contents
 	
  Small intestines and its contents
 	
  Large intestines and its contents
 	
  Liver
 	
  Gallbladder
  Spleen
 	
  Pancreas
  Kidneys and ureters
 	
  Urinary bladder
  Pelvic cavity	

____

Signature of the Doctor

____

* Injuries are to be given in serial number and mark them on the diagrams attached. In stab injuries, mention angles, margins and direction inside the body. In firearms injuries, mention direction and effects of fire.

Genital organs	
Spinal columns and spinal cord (opened where indicated)	

OPINION

a.   Probable time since death (keeping all factors including observations at inquest)

   i.   Between injury and death ____

   ii.   Between death and postmortem examination ____________________________

b.   Cause and manner of death. The cause of death to the best of my knowledge and belief is:

   i.   Immediate cause ____

   ii.   Due to ____

   iii.   Which of the injuries are antemortem/postmortem and duration if antemortem? _______________

   ____

   iv.   Manner of causation of injuries (if possible) ____________________________

   v.   Whether injuries (individually or collectively) are sufficient to cause death in ordinary course of nature or not? ____

c.   Any other ____

Specimens collected and preserved (*Tick '✓'*)

☐   Viscera (1. Stomach and small intestines with its contents, 2. Part of liver, half of each kidneys 3. Blood 4. Urine 5. Preservative used for sample 1 and 2, 6. Preservative used for sample 3 and 4)
☐   Sample of blood in gauze piece (dried)
☐   Clothes (air dried)
☐   Photographs/Video CD in case of custody deaths/Fingerprints
☐   Foreign body (like bullet, ligature)
☐   Slides from vagina or any other material ____________________________________
☐   Organs for histopathological examination

Place __________

____
Signature of the Doctor
Name (block letters), Designation and Seal

____

Received PM report No. ____________________________________ in original/copy along with body diagram and

____________________________ inquest papers (mention total number and initial them all).

(Viscera or any other specimen, if preserved is handed over to the police immediately after autopsy)

Name ____________________________ P.C. No. ____________________ P.S. ____________________

____
Signature and Date

Date _______________   **PM No.** _______________

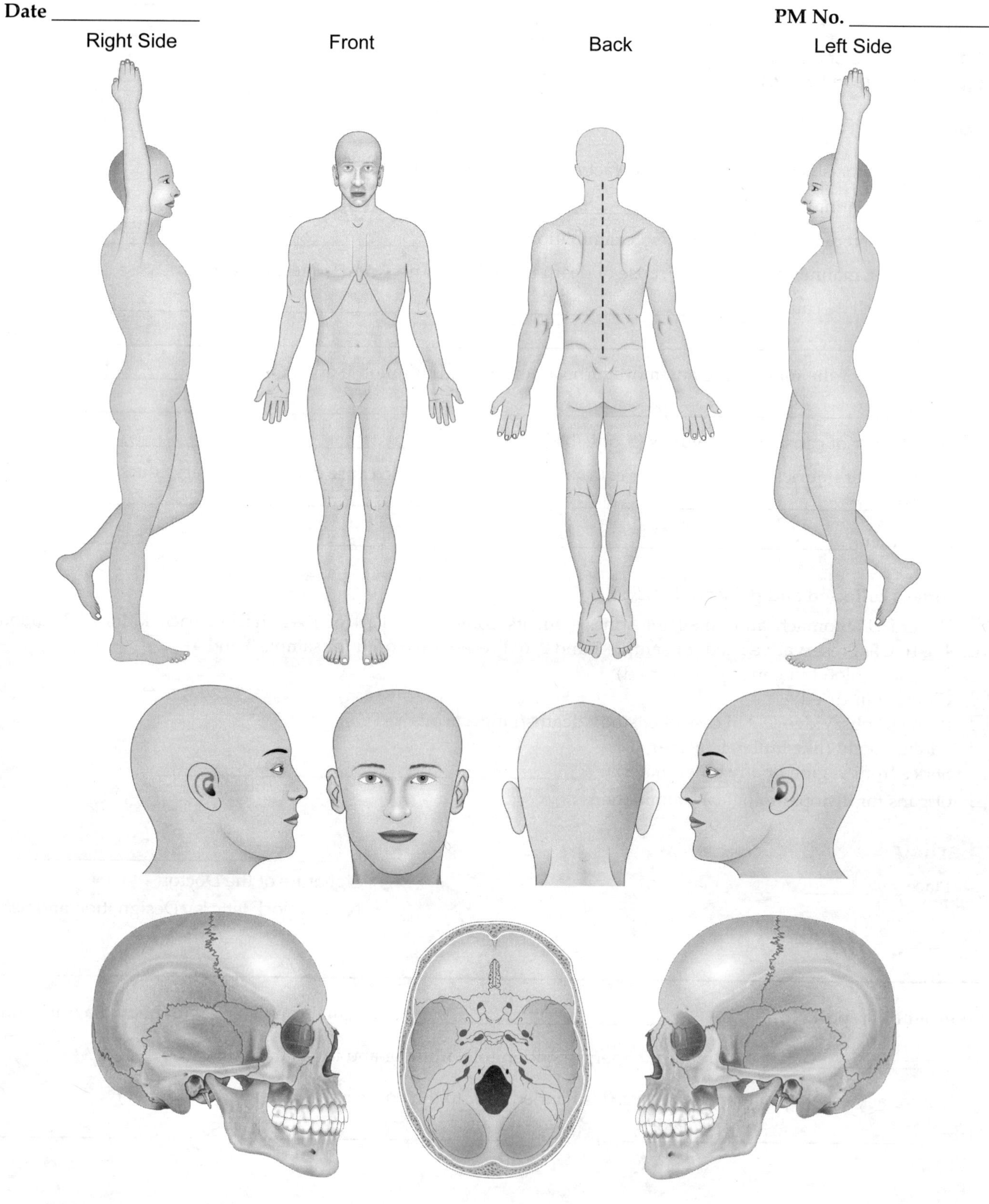

____
Signature of the Doctor
Name, Designation and Seal

EX. 6.4.4: POSTMORTEM REPORT

Department of Forensic Medicine and Toxicology

____

P.M. Report No. _____________________   C.R. No. __________________
(in case of hospital admission)

Date and time of receipt of body _____________________________

Date and time of receipt of inquest papers _________________

Date and time of commencement of autopsy _____________________

Time of completion of autopsy ___________ AM/PM

In case of hospital deaths (particular as per hospital records)

Date and time of admission _________________ Date and time of death __________________

Body brought by (Name, signature and rank/number of police official) _________________________________

____ Police Station __________________________________

Identified by (Name and addresses of relatives/persons acquainted along with their signature)

1. ____

2. ____

History (all events prior to death) ____

____

____

Information furnished by: ___________________________________

Particulars of Deceased

Name ___________________________________ Father's/Husband's name _______________________

Sex ___________________ Age ___________________ Race/Religion ______________________

Address ____

Identifications marks (if body is unidentified)

1. ____

2. ____

Height _____________ cm   Weight _____________ kg

Circumcision: Yes/No   Beard, mustache ___________________

____

Signature of the Doctor

SCHEDULE OF OBSERVATIONS

A. General	
Body	Entire and intact/Mutilated and in pieces
Clothings	
Medical intervention (if any)	
Built	Well/Moderate/Poor/Emaciated
Nourishment/Physique	Lean/Medium/Obese
Scars/Tattoos/Bedsores (if present)	
Skin	Pallor/Jaundiced/Pink/Cyanosis/Normal
Facial appearance	Pale/Normal/Livid/Cyanosed

Eyes
  Cornea
  Pupils
  Conjunctivae
	Closed/Half open/Open
	Clear/Hazy/Opaque　Arcus senilis: Absent/Developing/Fully developed
	Constricted/Dilated　Regular/Irregular
	Pale/Normal/Congested/Jaundiced/Hemorrhagic

Nostrils	
Ears	
Mouth	
Teeth	
Tongue	
Oral cavity	

Circum-oral regions
  Lips
  Inner aspects of lips
  Frenulum
	
	Pale/Cyanosed
	
	Intact/Torn

Orifice
  Urethral
  Anal
  Vaginal (in females)	

Condition of limbs	
Rigor mortis	Developing/Fully developed/Passing off　Mild/Strong
Postmortem staining	Fixed/Not fixed　　Areas present______

Decomposition changes
  Skin
  Face/Abdomen/Scrotum
  Foul smell
  Maggots
	
	Color changes of putrefaction/Marbling/Skin slippage
	Bloated/Not bloated
	Present/Absent
	Present/Absent

Any other findings	

Signature of the Doctor

B. External Injuries*
(Mention type, shape, length × breadth × depth of each injury and its relation to important body landmark. Indicate which injuries are fresh and which are old and their duration)

C. Internal Examination	

Head
  Scalp
  Skull
  Brain	

Neck	

Chest
  Ribs/Sternum/Chest wall
  Pleural cavities
  Lungs
    Right
    Left
  Pericardium
  Heart
    Coronaries
    Large blood vessels	

Abdomen
  Peritoneum
  Stomach and its contents
 	
  Small intestines and its contents
 	
  Large intestines and its contents
 	
  Liver
 	
  Gallbladder
  Spleen
 	
  Pancreas
  Kidneys and ureters
 	
  Urinary bladder
  Pelvic cavity	

Signature of the Doctor

* Injuries are to be given in serial number and mark them on the diagrams attached. In stab injuries, mention angles, margins and direction inside the body. In firearms injuries, mention direction and effects of fire.

Genital organs	
Spinal columns and spinal cord (opened where indicated)	

OPINION

a. Probable time since death (keeping all factors including observations at inquest)

    i. Between injury and death ____

    ii. Between death and postmortem examination ______________________________

b. Cause and manner of death. The cause of death to the best of my knowledge and belief is:

    i. Immediate cause ____

    ii. Due to ____

    iii. Which of the injuries are antemortem/postmortem and duration if antemortem? ________________

        ____

    iv. Manner of causation of injuries (if possible) ______________________________

    v. Whether injuries (individually or collectively) are sufficient to cause death in ordinary course of nature or not? ____

c. Any other ____

Specimens collected and preserved *(Tick '✓')*

☐ Viscera (1. Stomach and small intestines with its contents, 2. Part of liver, half of each kidneys 3. Blood 4. Urine 5. Preservative used for sample 1 and 2, 6. Preservative used for sample 3 and 4)

☐ Sample of blood in gauze piece (dried)

☐ Clothes (air dried)

☐ Photographs/Video CD in case of custody deaths/Fingerprints

☐ Foreign body (like bullet, ligature)

☐ Slides from vagina or any other material _______________________________________

☐ Organs for histopathological examination

Place __________

    ____
    Signature of the Doctor
    Name (block letters), Designation and Seal

Received PM report No. _______________________________________ in original/copy along with body diagram and

_______________________________ inquest papers (mention total number and initial them all).

(Viscera or any other specimen, if preserved is handed over to the police immediately after autopsy)

Name _______________________________ P.C. No. _______________________________ P.S. _______________________

____
Signature and Date

Date ______________   **PMR No.** ______________

| Right Side | Front | Back | Left Side |

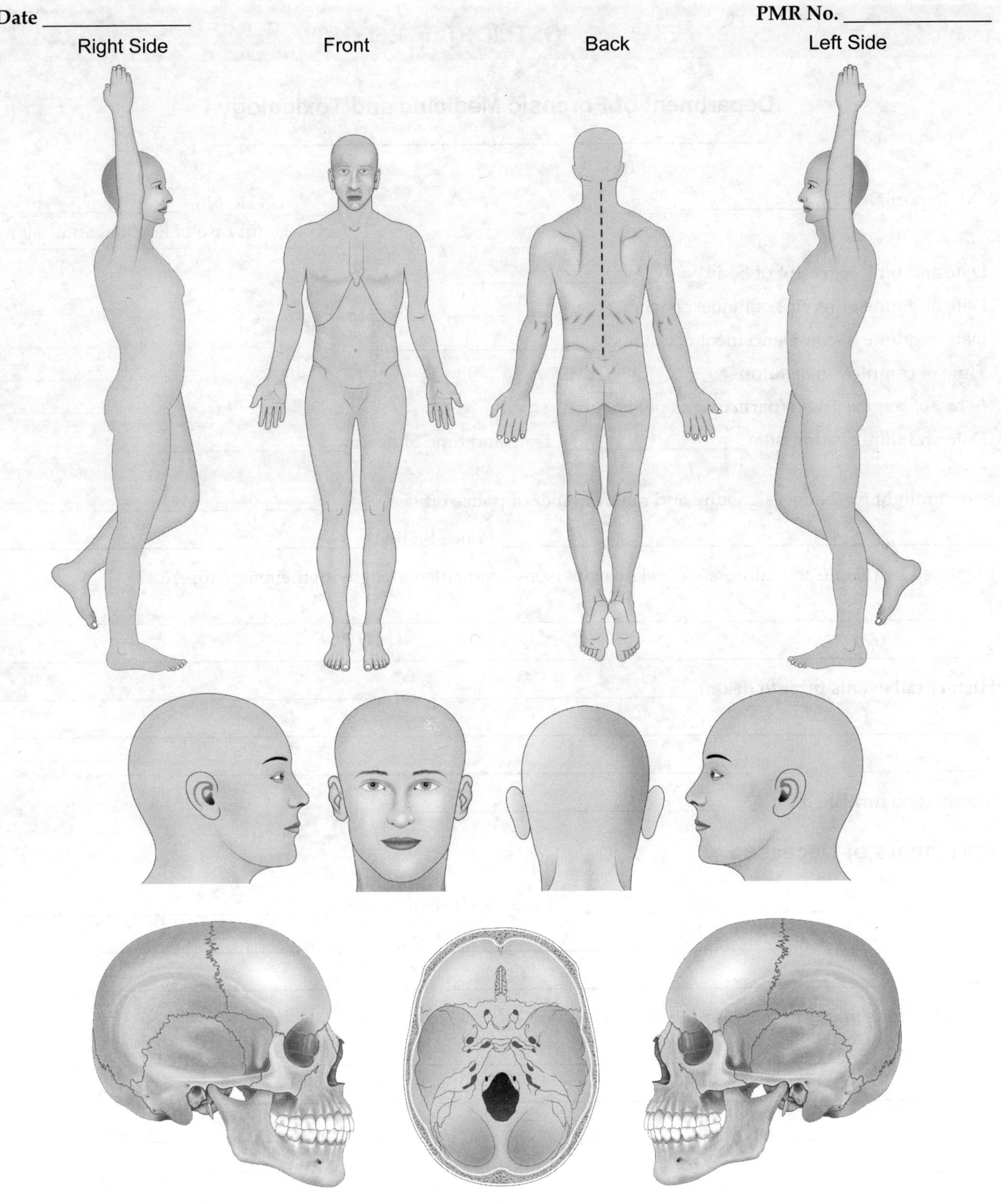

____
Signature of the Doctor
Name, Designation and Seal

EX. 6.4.5: POSTMORTEM REPORT

Department of Forensic Medicine and Toxicology

P.M. Report No. _______________   C.R. No. _______________
(in case of hospital admission)

Date and time of receipt of body _______________
Date and time of receipt of inquest papers _______________
Date and time of commencement of autopsy _______________
Time of completion of autopsy __________ AM/PM
In case of hospital deaths (particular as per hospital records)
Date and time of admission _______________ Date and time of death _______________

Body brought by (Name, signature and rank/number of police official) _______________
_______________ Police Station _______________

Identified by (Name and addresses of relatives/persons acquainted along with their signature)

1. _______________

2. _______________

History (all events prior to death) _______________

____

____

Information furnished by: _______________

Particulars of Deceased

Name _______________ Father's/Husband's name _______________

Sex _______________ Age _______________ Race/Religion _______________

Address _______________

Identifications marks (if body is unidentified)

1. _______________

2. _______________

Height __________ cm   Weight __________ kg

Circumcision: Yes/No   Beard, mustache _______________

____

Signature of the Doctor

SCHEDULE OF OBSERVATIONS

A. General	
Body	Entire and intact/Mutilated and in pieces
Clothings	
Medical intervention (if any)	
Built	Well/Moderate/Poor/Emaciated
Nourishment/Physique	Lean/Medium/Obese
Scars/Tattoos/Bedsores (if present)	
Skin	Pallor/Jaundiced/Pink/Cyanosis/Normal
Facial appearance	Pale/Normal/Livid/Cyanosed

Eyes
  Cornea
  Pupils
  Conjunctivae
	Closed/Half open/Open
	Clear/Hazy/Opaque Arcus senilis: Absent/Developing/Fully developed
	Constricted/Dilated Regular/Irregular
	Pale/Normal/Congested/Jaundiced/Hemorrhagic

Nostrils	
Ears	
Mouth	
Teeth	
Tongue	
Oral cavity	

Circum-oral regions
  Lips
  Inner aspects of lips
  Frenulum
	
	Pale/Cyanosed
	
	Intact/Torn

Orifice
  Urethral
  Anal
  Vaginal (in females)	

Condition of limbs	
Rigor mortis	Developing/Fully developed/Passing off Mild/Strong
Postmortem staining	Fixed/Not fixed Areas present________________

Decomposition changes
  Skin
  Face/Abdomen/Scrotum
  Foul smell
  Maggots
	
	Color changes of putrefaction/Marbling/Skin slippage
	Bloated/Not bloated
	Present/Absent
	Present/Absent

Any other findings	

Signature of the Doctor

B. External Injuries*
(Mention type, shape, length × breadth × depth of each injury and its relation to important body landmark. Indicate which injuries are fresh and which are old and their duration)

C. Internal Examination	

Head
  Scalp
  Skull
  Brain	

Neck	

Chest
  Ribs/Sternum/Chest wall
  Pleural cavities
  Lungs
    Right
    Left
  Pericardium
  Heart
    Coronaries
    Large blood vessels	

Abdomen
  Peritoneum
  Stomach and its contents
 	
  Small intestines and its contents
 	
  Large intestines and its contents
 	
  Liver
 	
  Gallbladder
  Spleen
 	
  Pancreas
  Kidneys and ureters
 	
  Urinary bladder
  Pelvic cavity	

Signature of the Doctor

* Injuries are to be given in serial number and mark them on the diagrams attached. In stab injuries, mention angles, margins and direction inside the body. In firearms injuries, mention direction and effects of fire.

Genital organs	
Spinal columns and spinal cord (opened where indicated)	

OPINION

a. Probable time since death (keeping all factors including observations at inquest)

    i. Between injury and death ____

    ii. Between death and postmortem examination _______________________________

b. Cause and manner of death. The cause of death to the best of my knowledge and belief is:

    i. Immediate cause ____

    ii. Due to ____

    iii. Which of the injuries are antemortem/postmortem and duration if antemortem? _______________

        ____

    iv. Manner of causation of injuries (if possible) _______________________________

    v. Whether injuries (individually or collectively) are sufficient to cause death in ordinary course of nature or not? ____

c. Any other ____

Specimens collected and preserved (*Tick '✓'*)

☐ Viscera (1. Stomach and small intestines with its contents, 2. Part of liver, half of each kidneys 3. Blood 4. Urine 5. Preservative used for sample 1 and 2, 6. Preservative used for sample 3 and 4)

☐ Sample of blood in gauze piece (dried)

☐ Clothes (air dried)

☐ Photographs/Video CD in case of custody deaths/Fingerprints

☐ Foreign body (like bullet, ligature)

☐ Slides from vagina or any other material ______________________________________

☐ Organs for histopathological examination

Place __________

                                       Signature of the Doctor
                                       Name (block letters), Designation and Seal

Received PM report No. ___________________________________ in original/copy along with body diagram and

___________________________ inquest papers (mention total number and initial them all).

(Viscera or any other specimen, if preserved is handed over to the police immediately after autopsy)

Name ___________________________________ P.C. No. ___________________________ P.S. ________________

                                        Signature and date

Date _______________   **PMR No.** _______________

| Right Side | Front | Back | Left Side |

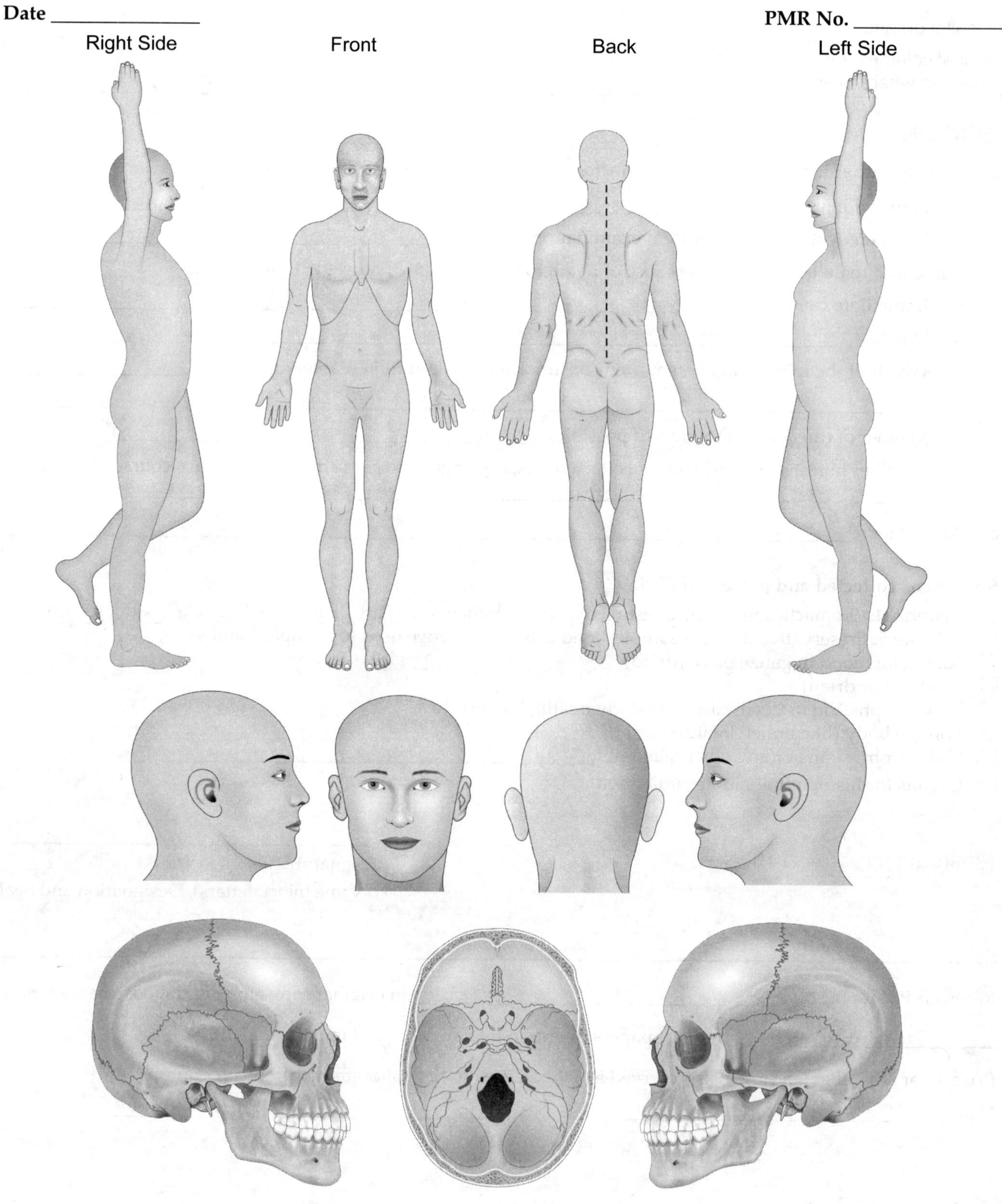

Signature of the Doctor
Name, Designation and Seal

EX. 6.4.6: POSTMORTEM REPORT

Department of Forensic Medicine and Toxicology

____

P.M. Report No. _________________________   C.R. No. _____________________
                                              (in case of hospital admission)

Date and time of receipt of body _______________________________

Date and time of receipt of inquest papers _________________

Date and time of commencement of autopsy ____________________________

Time of completion of autopsy ____________ AM/PM

In case of hospital deaths (particular as per hospital records)

Date and time of admission ___________________ Date and time of death _______________

Body brought by (Name, signature and rank/number of police official) _________________________________

____ Police Station ___________________________________

Identified by (Name and addresses of relatives/persons acquainted along with their signature)

1. ____

2. ____

History (all events prior to death) ____

____

____

Information furnished by: ____

Particulars of Deceased

Name ___________________________________ Father's/Husband's name ____________________________

Sex __________________________ Age ___________________ Race/Religion ______________________________

Address ____

Identifications marks (if body is unidentified)

1. ____

2. ____

Height ______________ cm   Weight _______________ kg

Circumcision: Yes/No   Beard, mustache __________________________

____

Signature of the Doctor

SCHEDULE OF OBSERVATIONS

A. General	
Body	Entire and intact/Mutilated and in pieces
Clothings	
Medical intervention (if any)	
Built	Well/Moderate/Poor/Emaciated
Nourishment/Physique	Lean/Medium/Obese
Scars/Tattoos/Bedsores (if present)	
Skin	Pallor/Jaundiced/Pink/Cyanosis/Normal
Facial appearance	Pale/Normal/Livid/Cyanosed

Eyes
  Cornea
  Pupils
  Conjunctivae
	Closed/Half open/Open
	Clear/Hazy/Opaque Arcus senilis: Absent/Developing/Fully developed
	Constricted/Dilated Regular/Irregular
	Pale/Normal/Congested/Jaundiced/Hemorrhagic

Nostrils	
Ears	
Mouth	
Teeth	
Tongue	
Oral cavity	

Circum-oral regions
  Lips
  Inner aspects of lips
  Frenulum
	Pale/Cyanosed
	
	Intact/Torn

Orifice
  Urethral
  Anal
  Vaginal (in females)	

Condition of limbs	
Rigor mortis	Developing/Fully developed/Passing off Mild/Strong
Postmortem staining	Fixed/Not fixed Areas present_______________________

Decomposition changes
  Skin
  Face/Abdomen/Scrotum
  Foul smell
  Maggots
	Color changes of putrefaction/Marbling/Skin slippage
	Bloated/Not bloated
	Present/Absent
	Present/Absent

Any other findings	

Signature of the Doctor

B. External Injuries*
(Mention type, shape, length × breadth × depth of each injury and its relation to important body landmark. Indicate which injuries are fresh and which are old and their duration)

C. Internal Examination	

Head
    Scalp
    Skull
    Brain	

Neck	

Chest
    Ribs/Sternum/Chest wall
    Pleural cavities
    Lungs
        Right
        Left
    Pericardium
    Heart
        Coronaries
        Large blood vessels	

Abdomen
    Peritoneum
 	
    Stomach and its contents
 	
    Small intestines and its contents
 	
    Large intestines and its contents
 	
    Liver
 	
    Gallbladder
    Spleen
 	
    Pancreas
    Kidneys and ureters
 	
    Urinary bladder
    Pelvic cavity	

Signature of the Doctor

---

* Injuries are to be given in serial number and mark them on the diagrams attached. In stab injuries, mention angles, margins and direction inside the body. In firearms injuries, mention direction and effects of fire.

Genital organs	
Spinal columns and spinal cord (opened where indicated)	

OPINION

a. Probable time since death (keeping all factors including observations at inquest)

    i.   Between injury and death ____

    ii. Between death and postmortem examination _______________________________

b. Cause and manner of death. The cause of death to the best of my knowledge and belief is:

    i.   Immediate cause ____

    ii. Due to ____

    iii. Which of the injuries are antemortem/postmortem and duration if antemortem? _______________

         ____

    iv. Manner of causation of injuries (if possible) ___________________________________

    v. Whether injuries (individually or collectively) are sufficient to cause death in ordinary course of nature or not? ____

c. Any other ____

Specimens collected and preserved *(Tick '✓')*

☐ Viscera (1. Stomach and small intestines with its contents, 2. Part of liver, half of each kidneys 3. Blood 4. Urine 5. Preservative used for sample 1 and 2, 6. Preservative used for sample 3 and 4)
☐ Sample of blood in gauze piece (dried)
☐ Clothes (air dried)
☐ Photographs/Video CD in case of custody deaths/Fingerprints
☐ Foreign body (like bullet, ligature)
☐ Slides from vagina or any other material _________________________________
☐ Organs for histopathological examination

Place __________   ________________________________

                                           Signature of the Doctor

                                         Name (block letters), Designation and Seal

Received PM report No. ________________________________ in original/copy along with body diagram and

________________________________ inquest papers (mention total number and initial them all).

(Viscera or any other specimen, if preserved is handed over to the police immediately after autopsy)

Name ________________________________ P.C. No. ________________________ P.S. ____________________

                                         Signature and Date

Date ________________

PMR No. ________________

Right Side   Front   Back   Left Side

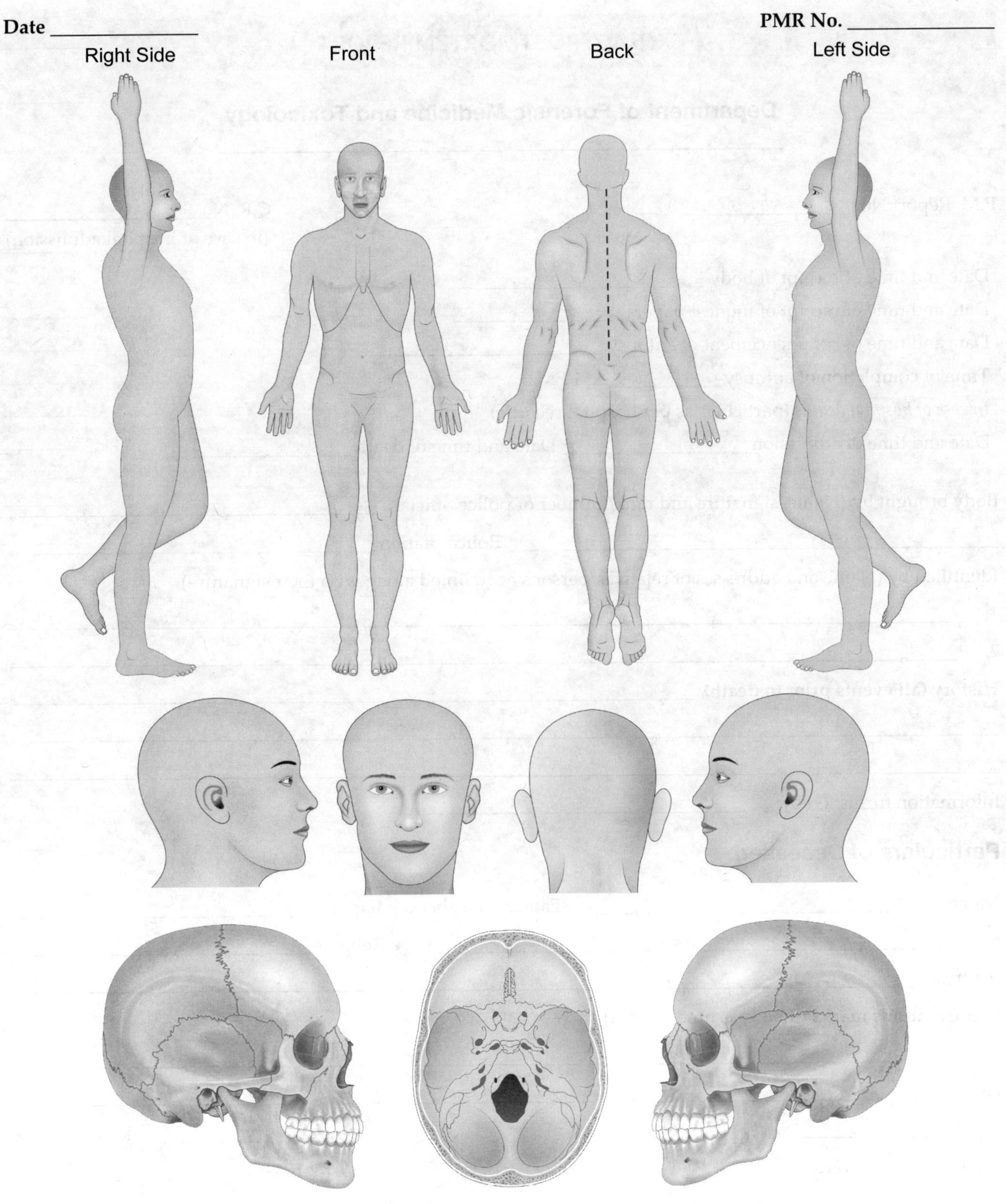

Signature of the Doctor
Name, Designation and Seal

EX. 6.4.7: POSTMORTEM REPORT

Department of Forensic Medicine and Toxicology

P.M. Report No. ________________

C.R. No. ________________
(in case of hospital admission)

Date and time of receipt of body ___________________

Date and time of receipt of inquest papers _______________

Date and time of commencement of autopsy ___________________

Time of completion of autopsy ___________ AM/PM

In case of hospital deaths (particular as per hospital records)

Date and time of admission ________________ Date and time of death _______________

Body brought by (Name, signature and rank/number of police official) ______________________________

____ Police Station _______________________________

Identified by (Name and addresses of relatives/persons acquainted along with their signature)

1. ____

2. ____

History (all events prior to death) ____

____

____

Information furnished by: __________________________________

Particulars of Deceased

Name ________________________________ Father's/Husband's name __________________________

Sex _________________________ Age __________________ Race/Religion _________________________

Address ____

Identifications marks (if body is unidentified)

1. ____

2. ____

Height _____________ cm

Weight _____________ kg

Circumcision: Yes/No

Beard, mustache ________________

____
Signature of the Doctor

SCHEDULE OF OBSERVATIONS

A. General	
Body	Entire and intact/Mutilated and in pieces
Clothings	
Medical intervention (if any)	
Built	Well/Moderate/Poor/Emaciated
Nourishment/Physique	Lean/Medium/Obese
Scars/Tattoos/Bedsores (if present)	
Skin	Pallor/Jaundiced/Pink/Cyanosis/Normal
Facial appearance	Pale/Normal/Livid/Cyanosed

Eyes
  Cornea
  Pupils
  Conjunctivae
	Closed/Half open/Open
	Clear/Hazy/Opaque Arcus senilis: Absent/Developing/Fully developed
	Constricted/Dilated Regular/Irregular
	Pale/Normal/Congested/Jaundiced/Hemorrhagic

Nostrils	
Ears	
Mouth	
Teeth	
Tongue	
Oral cavity	

Circum-oral regions
  Lips
  Inner aspects of lips
  Frenulum
	
	Pale/Cyanosed
	
	Intact/Torn

Orifice
  Urethral
  Anal
  Vaginal (in females)	

Condition of limbs	
Rigor mortis	Developing/Fully developed/Passing off Mild/Strong
Postmortem staining	Fixed/Not fixed Areas present_______________________

Decomposition changes
  Skin
  Face/Abdomen/Scrotum
  Foul smell
  Maggots
	
	Color changes of putrefaction/Marbling/Skin slippage
	Bloated/Not bloated
	Present/Absent
	Present/Absent

Any other findings	

Signature of the Doctor

<table>
<tr><td colspan="2" align="center">B. External Injuries*</td></tr>
<tr><td colspan="2">(Mention type, shape, length × breadth × depth of each injury and its relation to important body landmark. Indicate which injuries are fresh and which are old and their duration)</td></tr>
<tr><td colspan="2" align="center">C. Internal Examination</td></tr>
<tr><td>Head
  Scalp
  Skull
  Brain</td><td></td></tr>
<tr><td>Neck</td><td></td></tr>
<tr><td>Chest
  Ribs/Sternum/Chest wall
  Pleural cavities
  Lungs
    Right
    Left
  Pericardium
  Heart
    Coronaries
    Large blood vessels</td><td></td></tr>
<tr><td>Abdomen
  Peritoneum

  Stomach and its contents

  Small intestines and its contents

  Large intestines and its contents

  Liver

  Gallbladder
  Spleen

  Pancreas
  Kidneys and ureters

  Urinary bladder
  Pelvic cavity</td><td></td></tr>
</table>

Signature of the Doctor

* Injuries are to be given in serial number and mark them on the diagrams attached. In stab injuries, mention angles, margins and direction inside the body. In firearms injuries, mention direction and effects of fire.

Genital organs	
Spinal columns and spinal cord (opened where indicated)	

OPINION

a. Probable time since death (keeping all factors including observations at inquest)

   i.   Between injury and death ____

   ii. Between death and postmortem examination ___________________________________

b. Cause and manner of death. The cause of death to the best of my knowledge and belief is:

   i.   Immediate cause ____

   ii. Due to ____

   iii. Which of the injuries are antemortem/postmortem and duration if antemortem? _____________

   ____

   iv. Manner of causation of injuries (if possible) ________________________________

   v.   Whether injuries (individually or collectively) are sufficient to cause death in ordinary course of nature or not? ____

c. Any other ____

Specimens collected and preserved *(Tick '✓')*

☐ Viscera (1. Stomach and small intestines with its contents, 2. Part of liver, half of each kidneys 3. Blood 4. Urine 5. Preservative used for sample 1 and 2, 6. Preservative used for sample 3 and 4)
☐ Sample of blood in gauze piece (dried)
☐ Clothes (air dried)
☐ Photographs/Video CD in case of custody deaths/Fingerprints
☐ Foreign body (like bullet, ligature)
☐ Slides from vagina or any other material _________________________________
☐ Organs for histopathological examination

____

Place __________

Signature of the Doctor
Name (block letters), Designation and Seal

____

Received PM report No. ____________________________________ in original/copy along with body diagram and

____________________________ inquest papers (mention total number and initial them all).

(Viscera or any other specimen, if preserved is handed over to the police immediately after autopsy)

Name __________________________________ P.C. No. ___________________ P.S. _________________

____

Signature and Date

Date _______________   **PMR No.** _______________

| Right Side | Front | Back | Left Side |

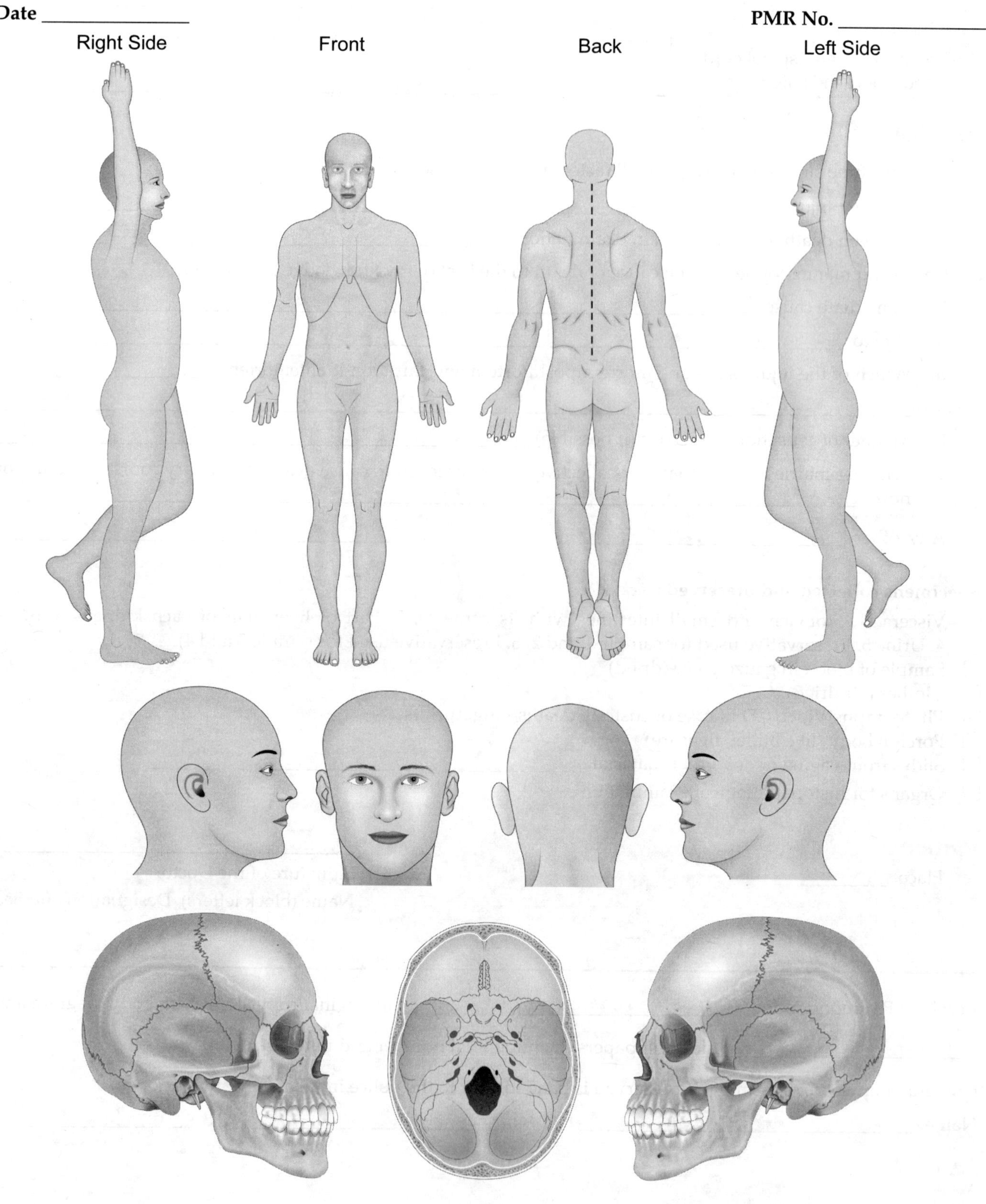

Signature of the Doctor
Name, Designation and Seal

EX. 6.4.8: POSTMORTEM REPORT

Department of Forensic Medicine and Toxicology

____

P.M. Report No. ________________   C.R. No. ________________
                                          (in case of hospital admission)

Date and time of receipt of body ______________________________

Date and time of receipt of inquest papers __________________

Date and time of commencement of autopsy ______________________

Time of completion of autopsy ____________ AM/PM

In case of hospital deaths (particular as per hospital records)

Date and time of admission __________________ Date and time of death __________________

Body brought by (Name, signature and rank/number of police official) ______________________________

____ Police Station ____________________________________

Identified by (Name and addresses of relatives/persons acquainted along with their signature)

1. ____

2. ____

History (all events prior to death) ____

____

____

Information furnished by: ____

Particulars of Deceased

Name _________________________________ Father's/Husband's name ______________________________

Sex ____________________________ Age ____________________ Race/Religion ____________________________

Address ____

Identifications marks (if body is unidentified)

1. ____

2. ____

Height ______________ cm   Weight ______________ kg

Circumcision: Yes/No   Beard, mustache __________________

____

Signature of the Doctor

SCHEDULE OF OBSERVATIONS

A. General	
Body	Entire and intact/Mutilated and in pieces
Clothings	
Medical intervention (if any)	
Built	Well/Moderate/Poor/Emaciated
Nourishment/Physique	Lean/Medium/Obese
Scars/Tattoos/Bedsores (if present)	
Skin	Pallor/Jaundiced/Pink/Cyanosis/Normal
Facial appearance	Pale/Normal/Livid/Cyanosed

Eyes
  Cornea
  Pupils
  Conjunctivae
	Closed/Half open/Open
	Clear/Hazy/Opaque Arcus senilis: Absent/Developing/Fully developed
	Constricted/Dilated Regular/Irregular
	Pale/Normal/Congested/Jaundiced/Hemorrhagic

Nostrils	
Ears	
Mouth	
Teeth	
Tongue	
Oral cavity	

Circum-oral regions
  Lips
  Inner aspects of lips
  Frenulum
	
	Pale/Cyanosed
	
	Intact/Torn

Orifice
  Urethral
  Anal
  Vaginal (in females)	

Condition of limbs	
Rigor mortis	Developing/Fully developed/Passing off Mild/Strong
Postmortem staining	Fixed/Not fixed Areas present_________________

Decomposition changes
  Skin
  Face/Abdomen/Scrotum
  Foul smell
  Maggots
	
	Color changes of putrefaction/Marbling/Skin slippage
	Bloated/Not bloated
	Present/Absent
	Present/Absent

Any other findings	

Signature of the Doctor

B. External Injuries*
(Mention type, shape, length × breadth × depth of each injury and its relation to important body landmark. Indicate which injuries are fresh and which are old and their duration)

C. Internal Examination	

Head
  Scalp
  Skull
  Brain	

Neck	

Chest
  Ribs/Sternum/Chest wall
  Pleural cavities
  Lungs
    Right
    Left
  Pericardium
  Heart
    Coronaries
    Large blood vessels	

Abdomen
  Peritoneum
 	
  Stomach and its contents
 	
  Small intestines and its contents
 	
  Large intestines and its contents
 	
  Liver
 	
  Gallbladder
  Spleen
 	
  Pancreas
  Kidneys and ureters
 	
  Urinary bladder
  Pelvic cavity	

Signature of the Doctor

* Injuries are to be given in serial number and mark them on the diagrams attached. In stab injuries, mention angles, margins and direction inside the body. In firearms injuries, mention direction and effects of fire.

Genital organs	
Spinal columns and spinal cord (opened where indicated)	

OPINION

a. Probable time since death (keeping all factors including observations at inquest)

  i.   Between injury and death ____

  ii. Between death and postmortem examination ______________________________

b. Cause and manner of death. The cause of death to the best of my knowledge and belief is:

  i.   Immediate cause ____

  ii. Due to ____

  iii. Which of the injuries are antemortem/postmortem and duration if antemortem? ____________

  ____

  iv. Manner of causation of injuries (if possible) ___________________________________

  v.   Whether injuries (individually or collectively) are sufficient to cause death in ordinary course of nature or not? ____

c. Any other ____

Specimens collected and preserved *(Tick '✓')*

☐ Viscera (1. Stomach and small intestines with its contents, 2. Part of liver, half of each kidneys 3. Blood 4. Urine 5. Preservative used for sample 1 and 2, 6. Preservative used for sample 3 and 4)
☐ Sample of blood in gauze piece (dried)
☐ Clothes (air dried)
☐ Photographs/Video CD in case of custody deaths/Fingerprints
☐ Foreign body (like bullet, ligature)
☐ Slides from vagina or any other material ___________________________________
☐ Organs for histopathological examination

Place __________   ________________________________

                                    Signature of the Doctor
                                    Name (block letters), Designation and Seal

____

Received PM report No. _________________________________ in original/copy along with body diagram and

_______________________ inquest papers (mention total number and initial them all).

(Viscera or any other specimen, if preserved is handed over to the police immediately after autopsy)

Name ___________________________ P.C. No. ___________________________ P.S. ___________________

                                    ____

                                    Signature and Date

Date _______________   PMR No. _______________

Right Side   Front   Back   Left Side

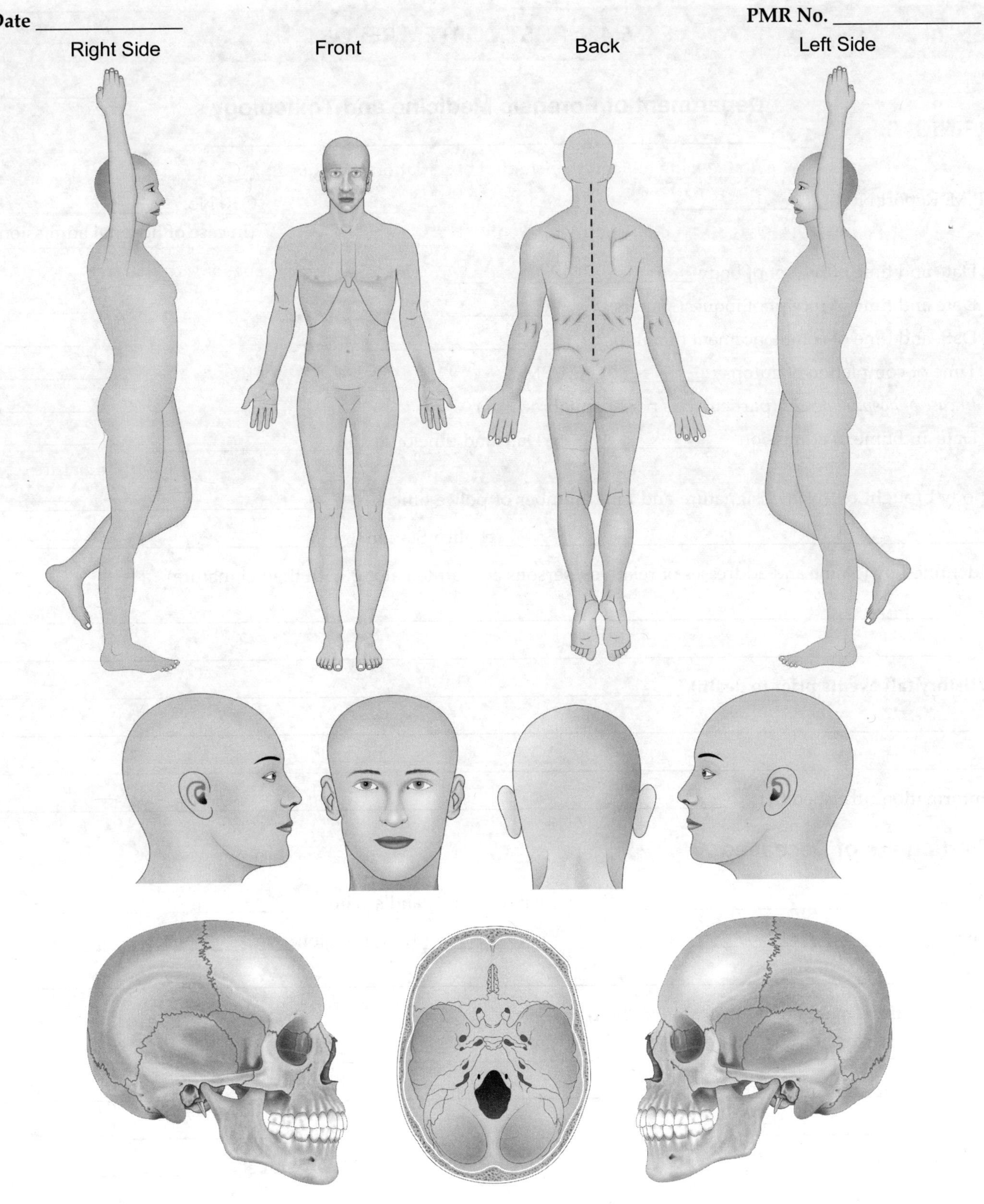

Signature of the Doctor
Name, Designation and Seal

EX. 6.4.9: POSTMORTEM REPORT

Department of Forensic Medicine and Toxicology

____

P.M. Report No. ________________   C.R. No. ___________________
                                          (in case of hospital admission)

Date and time of receipt of body ____________________

Date and time of receipt of inquest papers _______________

Date and time of commencement of autopsy ________________________

Time of completion of autopsy ___________ AM/PM

In case of hospital deaths (particular as per hospital records)

Date and time of admission ________________ Date and time of death ________________

Body brought by (Name, signature and rank/number of police official) ________________________________

____ Police Station ________________________________

Identified by (Name and addresses of relatives/persons acquainted along with their signature)

1. ____

2. ____

History (all events prior to death) ____

____

____

Information furnished by: ____

Particulars of Deceased

Name _______________________________ Father's/Husband's name ___________________________

Sex _____________________ Age _________________ Race/Religion ___________________________

Address ____

Identifications marks (if body is unidentified)

1. ____

2. ____

Height _____________ cm   Weight _____________ kg

Circumcision: Yes/No   Beard, mustache ___________________

____

Signature of the Doctor

SCHEDULE OF OBSERVATIONS

A. General	
Body	Entire and intact/Mutilated and in pieces
Clothings	
Medical intervention (if any)	
Built	Well/Moderate/Poor/Emaciated
Nourishment/Physique	Lean/Medium/Obese
Scars/Tattoos/Bedsores (if present)	
Skin	Pallor/Jaundiced/Pink/Cyanosis/Normal
Facial appearance	Pale/Normal/Livid/Cyanosed
Eyes 　Cornea 　Pupils 　Conjunctivae	Closed/Half open/Open Clear/Hazy/Opaque　　Arcus senilis: Absent/Developing/Fully developed Constricted/Dilated　　Regular/Irregular Pale/Normal/Congested/Jaundiced/Hemorrhagic
Nostrils	
Ears	
Mouth	
Teeth	
Tongue	
Oral cavity	
Circum-oral regions 　Lips 　Inner aspects of lips 　Frenulum	 Pale/Cyanosed Intact/Torn
Orifice 　Urethral 　Anal 　Vaginal (in females)	
Condition of limbs	
Rigor mortis	Developing/Fully developed/Passing off　　　　Mild/Strong
Postmortem staining	Fixed/Not fixed　　　　Areas present________________
Decomposition changes 　Skin 　Face/Abdomen/Scrotum 　Foul smell 　Maggots	 Color changes of putrefaction/Marbling/Skin slippage Bloated/Not bloated Present/Absent Present/Absent
Any other findings	

Signature of the Doctor

B. External Injuries*
(Mention type, shape, length × breadth × depth of each injury and its relation to important body landmark. Indicate which injuries are fresh and which are old and their duration)

C. Internal Examination	

Head
  Scalp
  Skull
  Brain	

Neck	

Chest
  Ribs/Sternum/Chest wall
  Pleural cavities
  Lungs
    Right
    Left
  Pericardium
  Heart
    Coronaries
    Large blood vessels	

Abdomen
  Peritoneum
 	
  Stomach and its contents
 	
  Small intestines and its contents
 	
  Large intestines and its contents
 	
  Liver
 	
  Gallbladder
  Spleen
 	
  Pancreas
  Kidneys and ureters
 	
  Urinary bladder
  Pelvic cavity	

Signature of the Doctor

* Injuries are to be given in serial number and mark them on the diagrams attached. In stab injuries, mention angles, margins and direction inside the body. In firearms injuries, mention direction and effects of fire.

Genital organs	
Spinal columns and spinal cord (opened where indicated)	

OPINION

a. Probable time since death (keeping all factors including observations at inquest)

    i.   Between injury and death ____

    ii. Between death and postmortem examination _________________________________

b. Cause and manner of death. The cause of death to the best of my knowledge and belief is:

    i.   Immediate cause ____

    ii. Due to ____

    iii. Which of the injuries are antemortem/postmortem and duration if antemortem? __________

       ____

    iv. Manner of causation of injuries (if possible) ________________________________

    v. Whether injuries (individually or collectively) are sufficient to cause death in ordinary course of nature or not? ____

c. Any other ____

Specimens collected and preserved *(Tick '✓')*

☐ Viscera (1. Stomach and small intestines with its contents, 2. Part of liver, half of each kidneys 3. Blood 4. Urine 5. Preservative used for sample 1 and 2, 6. Preservative used for sample 3 and 4)
☐ Sample of blood in gauze piece (dried)
☐ Clothes (air dried)
☐ Photographs/Video CD in case of custody deaths/Fingerprints
☐ Foreign body (like bullet, ligature)
☐ Slides from vagina or any other material _______________________________________
☐ Organs for histopathological examination

Place ___________   _______________________________

                                                    Signature of the Doctor

                                                    Name (block letters), Designation and Seal

---

Received PM report No. ______________________________________ in original/copy along with body diagram and

_______________________________ inquest papers (mention total number and initial them all).

(Viscera or any other specimen, if preserved is handed over to the police immediately after autopsy)

Name ___________________________________ P.C. No. ______________________________ P.S. ___________________

                                                    ____

                                                    Signature and Date

Date _______________   **PMR No.** _______________

| Right Side | Front | Back | Left Side |

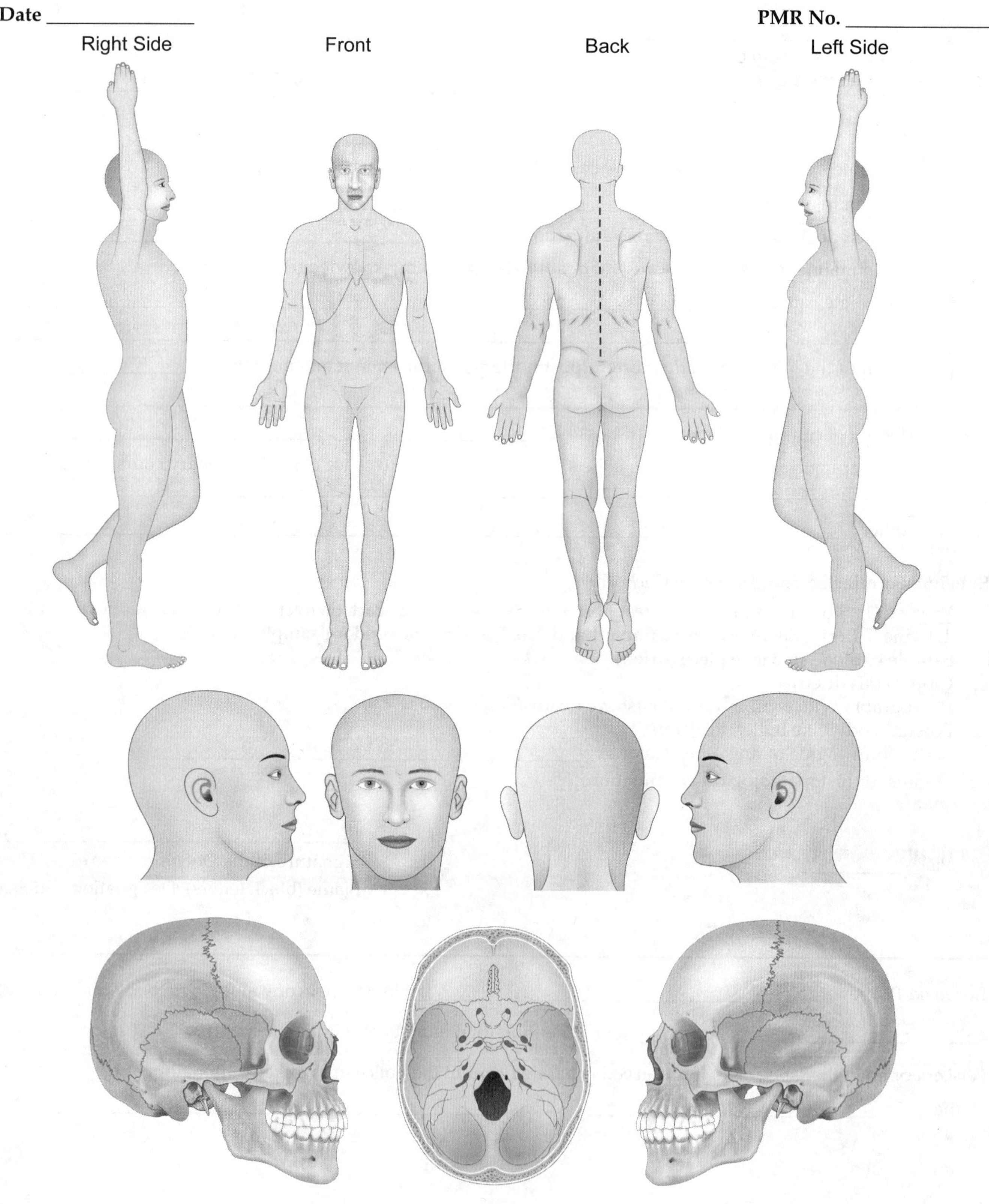

Signature of the Doctor
Name, Designation and Seal

EX. 6.4.10: POSTMORTEM REPORT

Department of Forensic Medicine and Toxicology

____

P.M. Report No. _________________

C.R. No. _________________
(in case of hospital admission)

Date and time of receipt of body _____________________

Date and time of receipt of inquest papers _______________

Date and time of commencement of autopsy _________________

Time of completion of autopsy ___________ AM/PM

In case of hospital deaths (particular as per hospital records)

Date and time of admission _________________ Date and time of death _________________

Body brought by (Name, signature and rank/number of police official) _________________

_______________________________________ Police Station _________________________________

Identified by (Name and addresses of relatives/persons acquainted along with their signature)

1. ____

2. ____

History (all events prior to death) ____

____

____

Information furnished by: ____

Particulars of Deceased

Name _________________________________ Father's/Husband's name _________________________

Sex _________________________ Age _________________ Race/Religion _________________________

Address ____

Identifications marks (if body is unidentified)

1. ____

2. ____

Height _____________ cm

Weight _____________ kg

Circumcision: Yes/No

Beard, mustache _________________

____

Signature of the Doctor

SCHEDULE OF OBSERVATIONS

A. General	
Body	Entire and intact/Mutilated and in pieces
Clothings	
Medical intervention (if any)	
Built	Well/Moderate/Poor/Emaciated
Nourishment/Physique	Lean/Medium/Obese
Scars/Tattoos/Bedsores (if present)	
Skin	Pallor/Jaundiced/Pink/Cyanosis/Normal
Facial appearance	Pale/Normal/Livid/Cyanosed

Eyes
  Cornea
  Pupils
  Conjunctivae
	Closed/Half open/Open
	Clear/Hazy/Opaque Arcus senilis: Absent/Developing/Fully developed
	Constricted/Dilated Regular/Irregular
	Pale/Normal/Congested/Jaundiced/Hemorrhagic

Nostrils	
Ears	
Mouth	
Teeth	
Tongue	
Oral cavity	

Circum-oral regions
  Lips
  Inner aspects of lips
  Frenulum
	
	Pale/Cyanosed
	
	Intact/Torn

Orifice
  Urethral
  Anal
  Vaginal (in females)	

Condition of limbs	
Rigor mortis	Developing/Fully developed/Passing off Mild/Strong
Postmortem staining	Fixed/Not fixed Areas present_____________________

Decomposition changes
  Skin
  Face/Abdomen/Scrotum
  Foul smell
  Maggots
	
	Color changes of putrefaction/Marbling/Skin slippage
	Bloated/Not bloated
	Present/Absent
	Present/Absent

Any other findings	

Signature of the Doctor

B. External Injuries*
(Mention type, shape, length × breadth × depth of each injury and its relation to important body landmark. Indicate which injuries are fresh and which are old and their duration)

C. Internal Examination	

Head
  Scalp
  Skull
  Brain	

Neck	

Chest
  Ribs/Sternum/Chest wall
  Pleural cavities
  Lungs
    Right
    Left
  Pericardium
  Heart
    Coronaries
    Large blood vessels	

Abdomen
  Peritoneum
 	
  Stomach and its contents
 	
  Small intestines and its contents
 	
  Large intestines and its contents
 	
  Liver
 	
  Gallbladder
  Spleen
 	
  Pancreas
  Kidneys and ureters
 	
  Urinary bladder
  Pelvic cavity	

Signature of the Doctor

* Injuries are to be given in serial number and mark them on the diagrams attached. In stab injuries, mention angles, margins and direction inside the body. In firearms injuries, mention direction and effects of fire.

Genital organs	
Spinal columns and spinal cord (opened where indicated)	

OPINION

a. Probable time since death (keeping all factors including observations at inquest)

    i.   Between injury and death ____

    ii.   Between death and postmortem examination ____________________________

b. Cause and manner of death. The cause of death to the best of my knowledge and belief is:

    i.   Immediate cause ____

    ii.   Due to ____

    iii. Which of the injuries are antemortem/postmortem and duration if antemortem? ____________________

          ____

    iv. Manner of causation of injuries (if possible) _____________________________

    v.   Whether injuries (individually or collectively) are sufficient to cause death in ordinary course of nature or not? ____

c. Any other ____

Specimens collected and preserved (*Tick '✓'*)

☐ Viscera (1. Stomach and small intestines with its contents, 2. Part of liver, half of each kidneys 3. Blood 4. Urine 5. Preservative used for sample 1 and 2, 6. Preservative used for sample 3 and 4)
☐ Sample of blood in gauze piece (dried)
☐ Clothes (air dried)
☐ Photographs/Video CD in case of custody deaths/Fingerprints
☐ Foreign body (like bullet, ligature)
☐ Slides from vagina or any other material ___________________________________
☐ Organs for histopathological examination

    Place __________   _______________________________

                                       Signature of the Doctor

                                     Name (block letters), Designation and Seal

---

Received PM report No. _____________________________ in original/copy along with body diagram and

_______________________ inquest papers (mention total number and initial them all).

(Viscera or any other specimen, if preserved is handed over to the police immediately after autopsy)

Name ______________________ P.C. No. ______________________ P.S. ______________________

                                        ____

                                        Signature and Date

Date _______________ **PMR No.** _______________

| Right Side | Front | Back | Left Side |

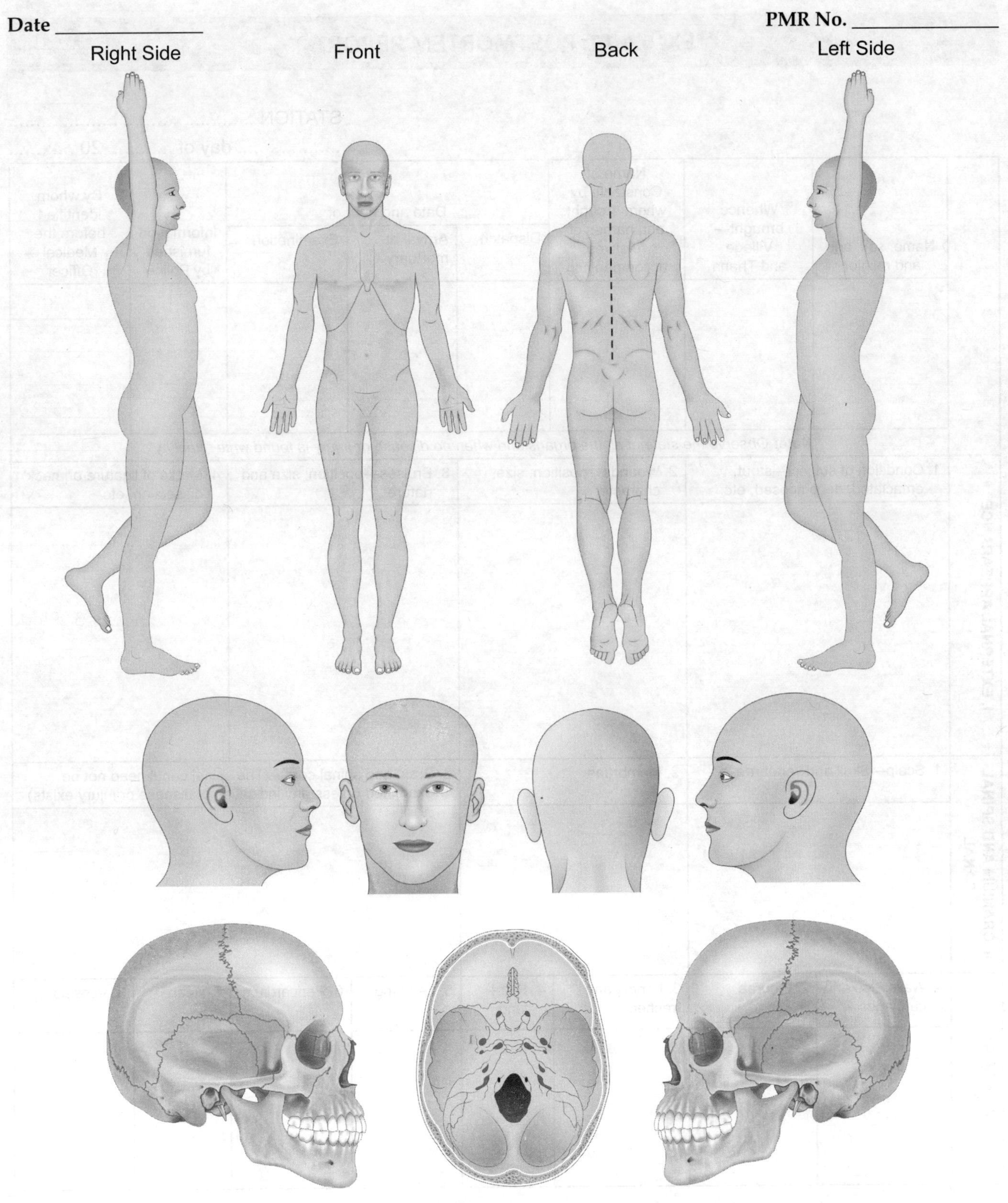

____
Signature of the Doctor
Name, Designation and Seal

EX. 6.4.11: POSTMORTEM REPORT

STATION ....

.... day of .... 20 ....

	Name, sex, age and religion	Whence brought— Village and Thana	Name of Constable by whom brought and names of relatives accompanying	Date and hour of			Information furnished by Police	By whom identified before the Medical Officer
				Dispatch	Arrival at mortuary	Examination		

Note: *Observe the state of all the organs and when no disease or injury is found write "Healthy"*

I. EXTERNAL APPEARANCE	1. Condition of subject—stout, emaciated, decomposed, etc.	2. Wounds—position, size, character	3. Bruises—position, size and nature	4. Marks of ligature on neck, dissection, etc.

II. CRANIUM AND SPINAL CANAL	1. Scalp—Skull and vertebrae	2. Membrane	3. Brain and spinal cord—(The spinal canal need not be examined unless any indication of disease or injury exists)

III. THORAX	1. Walls, ribs and cartilages	2. Pleurae	3. Larynx and trachea	4. Right lung	5. Left lung	6. Pericardium	7. Heart	8. Vessels

(Contd...)

(Contd...)

	1. Walls	2. Peritoneum	3. Mouth, pharynx and esophagus	4. Stomach and its contents	5. Small intestine and its contents	6. Large intestine and its contents
IV. ABDOMEN						
	7. Liver	8. Spleen	9. Kidneys	10. Bladder	11. Organs of generation, external and internal	

	1. Injury	2. Disease or deformity	3. Fracture	4. Dislocation
MUSCLES, BONES AND JOINTS				

MORE DETAILED DESCRIPTION OF INJURY OR DISEASE

OPINION OF THE MEDICAL OFFICER AS TO THE CAUSE OF DEATH AND TIME SINCE DEATH	REMARKS BY CIVIL SURGEON
Note: In the case of wounded note whether there is any indication of the wounds being homicidal, suicidal or otherwise. Assistant Surgeon of	Civil Surgeon of .... The .... day of ....20............

Date _____________   **PMR No.** _____________

| Right Side | Front | Back | Left Side |

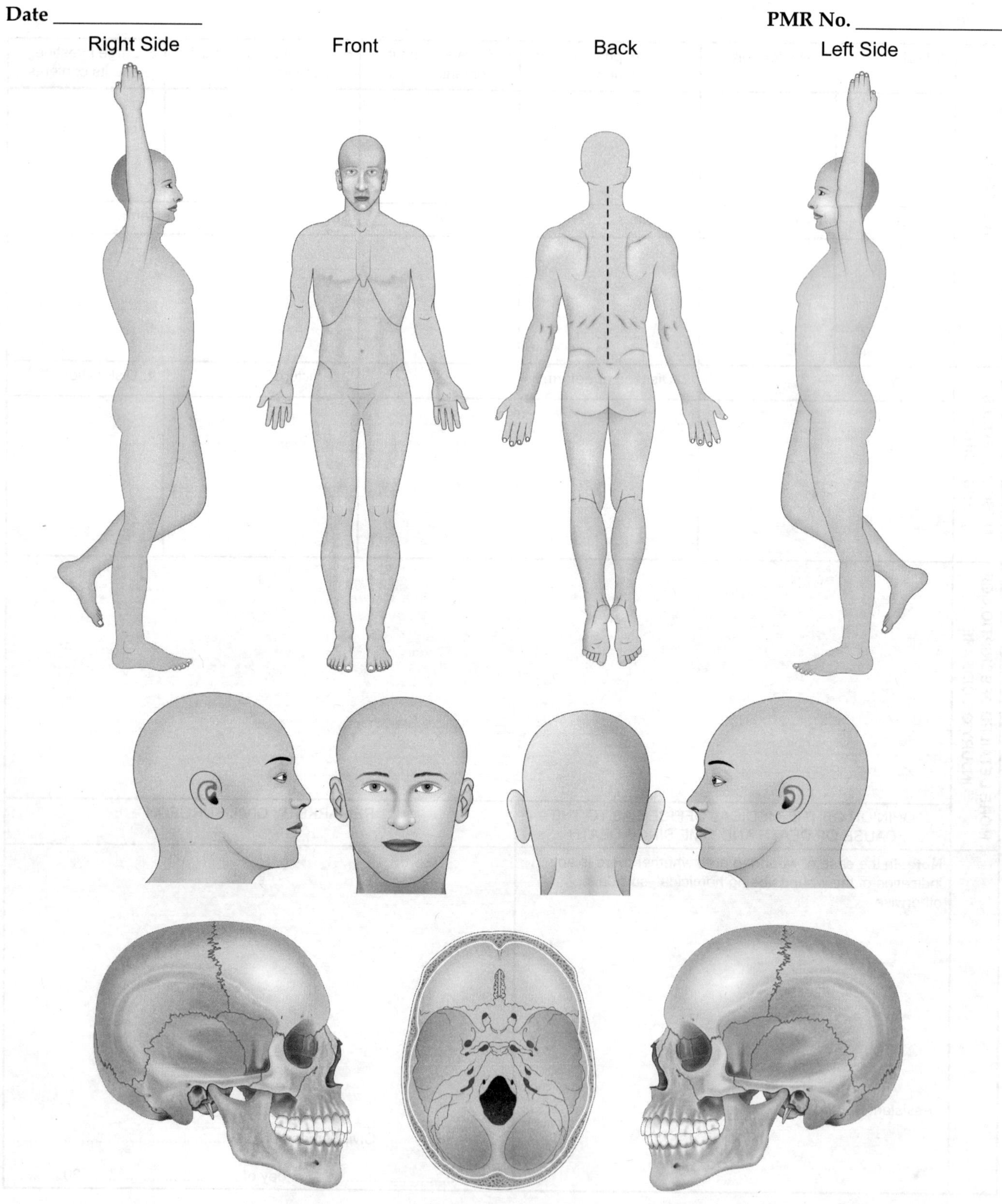

Signature of the Doctor
Name, Designation and Seal

EX. 6.4.12: POSTMORTEM REPORT

REPORT OF POSTMORTEM EXAMINATION

On the body of ____

Place __________________   Date __________________   Time __________

Body identified by Police Constable and Choukidar

Probable age

Probable time since death

A–EXTERNAL EXAMINATION

1. Condition of body as regards muscularity, stoutness, emaciation, rigor mortis and decomposition.

____

2. Marks of identification, especially in the case of the body of an unknown person.

____

3. Eyes

____

4. State of natural orifices, ears nostrils, mouth, anus, urethra, vagina.

____

5. Injuries—natural, exact position and measurements including direction especially in incised wounds.

____

____

____

____

____

6. Bones and joints

____

7. External organs of generation

____

8. Additional remarks

____

B–INTERNAL EXAMINATION
I–HEAD AND NECK

1. Scalp, Skull Bones (Vertex)

2. Membranes

3. Brain

4. Base of Skull

5. Vertebrae

6. Spinal cord

7. Additional remarks

Spinal cord need not be examined unless any indications of disease, strychnine poisoning or injury exist.

II–THORAX

1. Walls, ribs, cartilages

2. Pleurae

3. Larynx, trachea and bronchi

4. Right-lung

5. Left-lung

6. Pericardium

7. Heart with weight

8. Large vessels

9. Additional remarks

III–ABDOMEN

1. Walls

2. Peritoneum

3. Cavity

4. Buccal cavity, teeth, tongue and pharynx

5. Esophagus

6. Stomach and its contents

7. Small intestine and its contents

8. Large intestines and its contents

9. Liver (with weight) and gallbladder

10. Pancreas

11. Spleen with weight

12. Kidneys with weight

13. Bladder

14. Organs of generation

15. Additional remarks wherever possible. Medical Officer's deduction from the state of the contents of the stomach as to time of death and last meal.

C. Date and hour of onset of symptoms   To be answered in case of poisoning

Date and hour of death

D. Opinion as to cause and manner of death

Place _______________

Date _______________   Medical Officer _______________

In case of exhumation, the dates of burial and exhumation should be furnished.

REMARKS BY CIVIL SURGEON

Place _______________

Date _______________   Civil Surgeon of _______________

Date _______________   **PMR No.** _______________

| Right Side | Front | Back | Left Side |

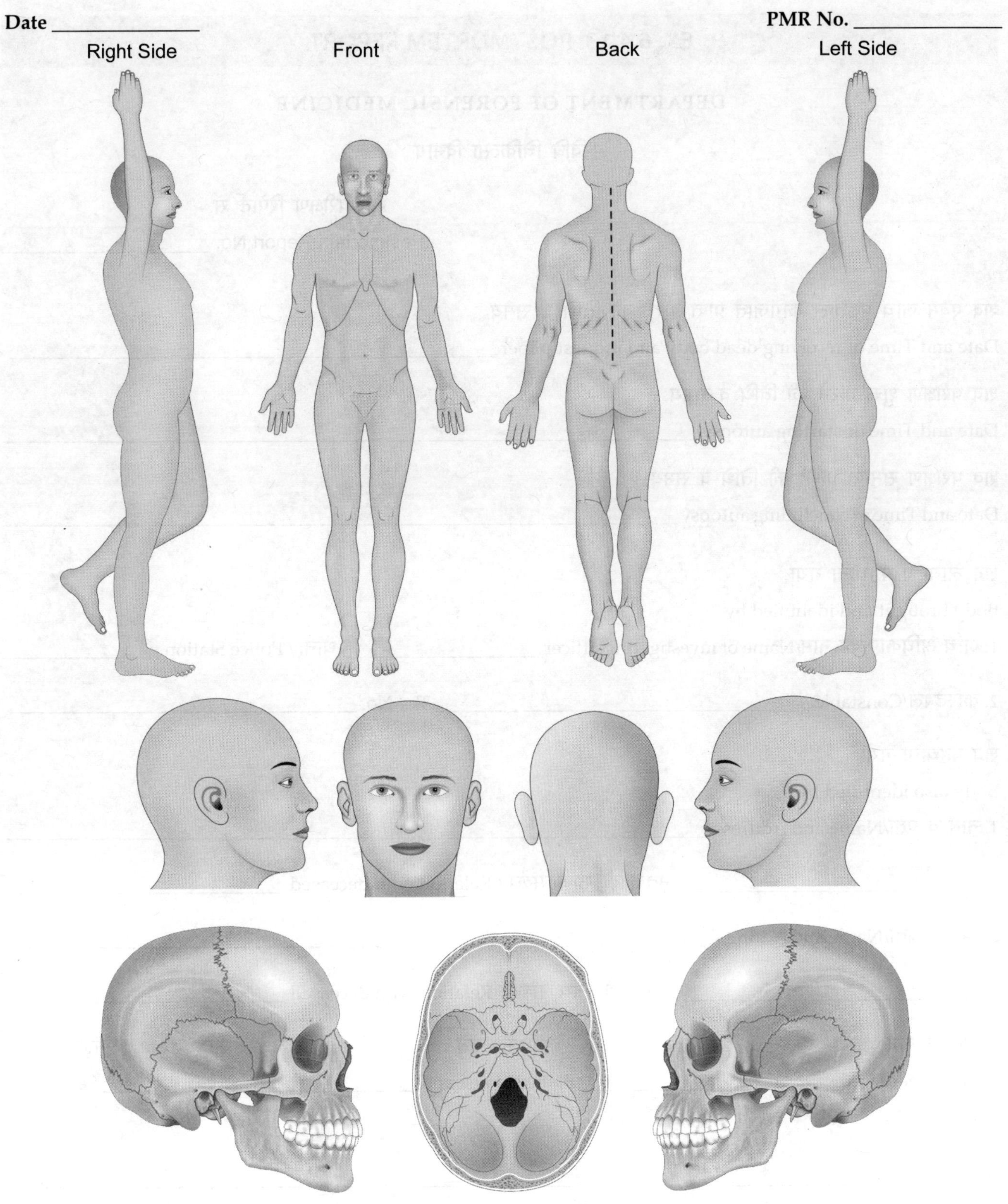

____
Signature of the Doctor
Name, Designation and Seal

EX. 6.4.13: POSTMORTEM REPORT

DEPARTMENT OF FORENSIC MEDICINE

विधि चिकित्सा विभाग

शव परीक्षण रिपोर्ट सं.

Postmortem Report No. ___________________

शव एवम जांच पड़ताल कागजात प्राप्त करने की तिथि व समय

Date and Time of receiving dead body and inquest paper ___________________________________

शव परीक्षण शुरू करने की तिथि व समय

Date and Time of starting autopsy ___________________________________

शव परीक्षण समाप्त करने की तिथि व समय

Date and Time of concluding autopsy ___________________________________

शव लाया व पहचाना गया

Body brought and identified by

1. जांच अधिकार का नाम/Name of investigating officer _________________ थाना / Police Station ____________

2. कांस्टेबल/Constable _________________________ सं. / No. _____________________

शव पहचाना गया

Body also identified by

1. नाम व पता/Name and Address ___________________________________

___________________________ मृतक के साथ संबंध / Relation with deceased ______________________

2. नाम व पता/Name and Address ___________________________________

___________________________ मृतक के साथ संबंध / Relation with deceased ______________________

मृतक का नाम	पिता / पति	आयु	लिंग
Name of deceased _______________	Father / Husband _____________	Age _______	Sex _______

पता

Address ___________________________________

मामले का संक्षिप्त इतिवृत (जांच पडताल कागजातों के अनुसार)

Brief history of the case (As per Inquest Paper)___________________________________

उँचाई/Height _________________________________   भार/Weight _________________________

शव परीक्षण रिपोर्ट सं.
Postmortem Report No._________________________

(क) सामान्य अवलोकन

(A) General Observation

(ख) बाहय चोटों का विवरण

(B) Details of External Injuries

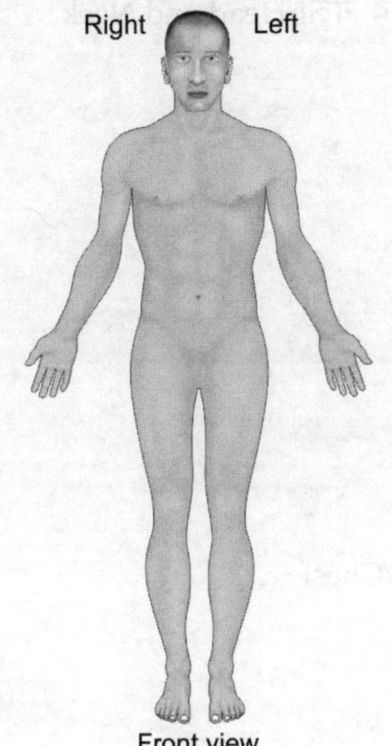

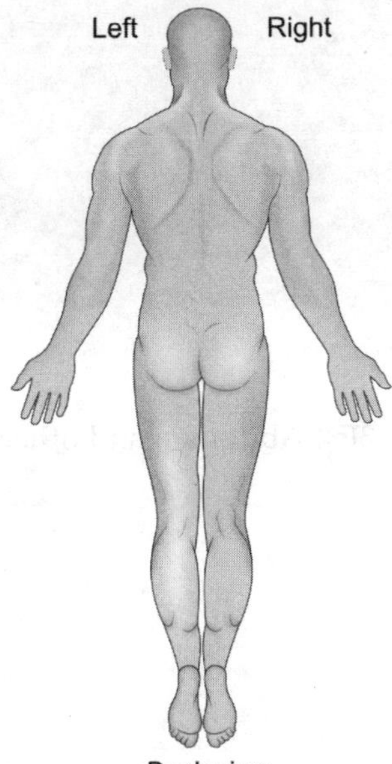

शव परीक्षण रिपोर्ट सं.

Postmortem Report No. _______________________

(ग) आन्तरिक परीक्षण
(C) Internal Examinations

1. सिर व गला/Head and Neck

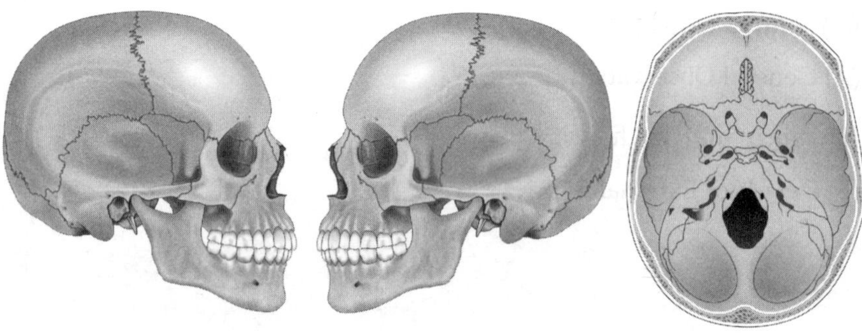

Right lateral view   Left lateral view   Base of skull

2. छाती/Chest

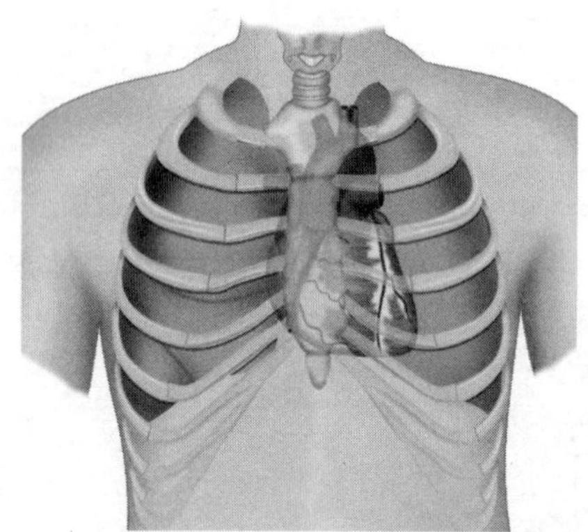

3. पेट व अन्य/Abdomen and others

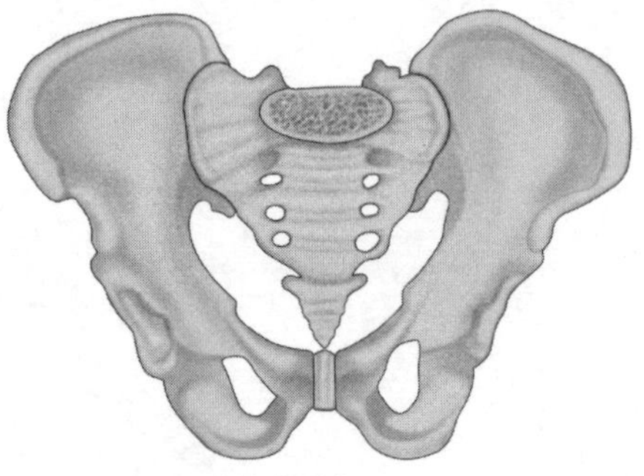

Pelvis

शव परीक्षण रिपोर्ट सं.

Postmortem Report No. _______________________

(घ) रासायनिक विश्लेषण के लिए रखे गए सुरक्षित नमुने (यदि आवश्यक हो)

(D) Viscera preserved for chemical analysis during autopsy (if required) _______________________

(ड) परिरक्षी प्रयोग में लाया गया

(E) Preservative used—Saturated solution or common salt/rectified spirit any other _______________________

(च) कपडे /अन्य सुरक्षित रखी गई वस्तुएं (यदि कोई हों)

(F) Clothes/other articles preserved during autopsy (if any) _______________________

(छ) टिप्पणियों (यदि कोई हो)

(H) Remarks (if any) _______________________

(ज) निष्कर्ष

(G) Opinion _______________________

चिकित्सा अधिकारी का पद नाम व हस्ताक्षर

Signature and Designation of Medical Officer

पुलिस को दी गई वस्तुएं:

Item handed over to police

1. जांच पड़ताल के कागजात/Inquest Papers _______________________ in numbers.

2. शव परिक्षण/Postmortem report in original

प्राप्तकर्ता पुलिस जांच अधिकारी का नाम   सं.   पुलिस स्टेशन

Name of receiving police/investigating officer   No.   Police Station

हस्ताक्षर

Signature

EX. 6.4.14: POSTMORTEM REPORT

Department of Forensic Medicine and Toxicology

P.M. No./ ________________   Place: ___________________

                                                                 Date: __________________

Name: ___________________________________ Sex: _________ Age: _________ Caste and Religion: ____________

Police station: ____

UDR No.: ___________________________________ Under section: _________________________________

Body identified by: _________________________________ Name: ___________________________

Police station: ____

Date and hour of receipt of requisition: ____

Date and hour of examination: ____

Date and hour of dispatch: ____

INFORMATION FURNISHED BY THE POLICE

____

____

As per the information furnished by police in Form No. 146 (i) (ii),

____

(I) External Examination
(Condition of subject, wounds position, size and character)

(II) Cranium, Spinal Canal and Neck Structures

1. Scalp:
2. Skull:
3. Vertebral column:
4. Brain:
5. Spinal cord:
6. Neck structures:

(III) Thorax
1. Walls, ribs and cartilages:
2. Pleurae and pleural cavity:
3. Trachea and larynx:
4. Right lung:
5. Left lung:
6. Pericardium:
7. Heart:
8. Coronaries:
9. Large vessels:

(IV) Abdomen
1. Walls:
2. Peritoneum:
3. Mouth, pharynx and esophagus:
4. Diaphragm:
5. Stomach and its contents:
6. Small intestine and its contents:
7. Large intestine and its contents:
8. Liver:
9. Spleen:
10. Adrenals:
11. Pancreas:

(V) Genito-Urinary Organs
1. Kidneys:
2. Bladder:
3. Organs of generation:

OTHER RELEVANT INFORMATION

____

____

Investigations:

1. Blood and Viscera sent to FSL:

2. Histopathology—Heart, Brain, Lungs, Liver, Kidney and Spleen:

____

OPINION AS TO CAUSE OF DEATH

____

____

Place: ___________________

Date: ___________________

                     ____

                     Doctor's Signature

Date _______________

PM No. _______________

Right Side	Front	Back	Left Side

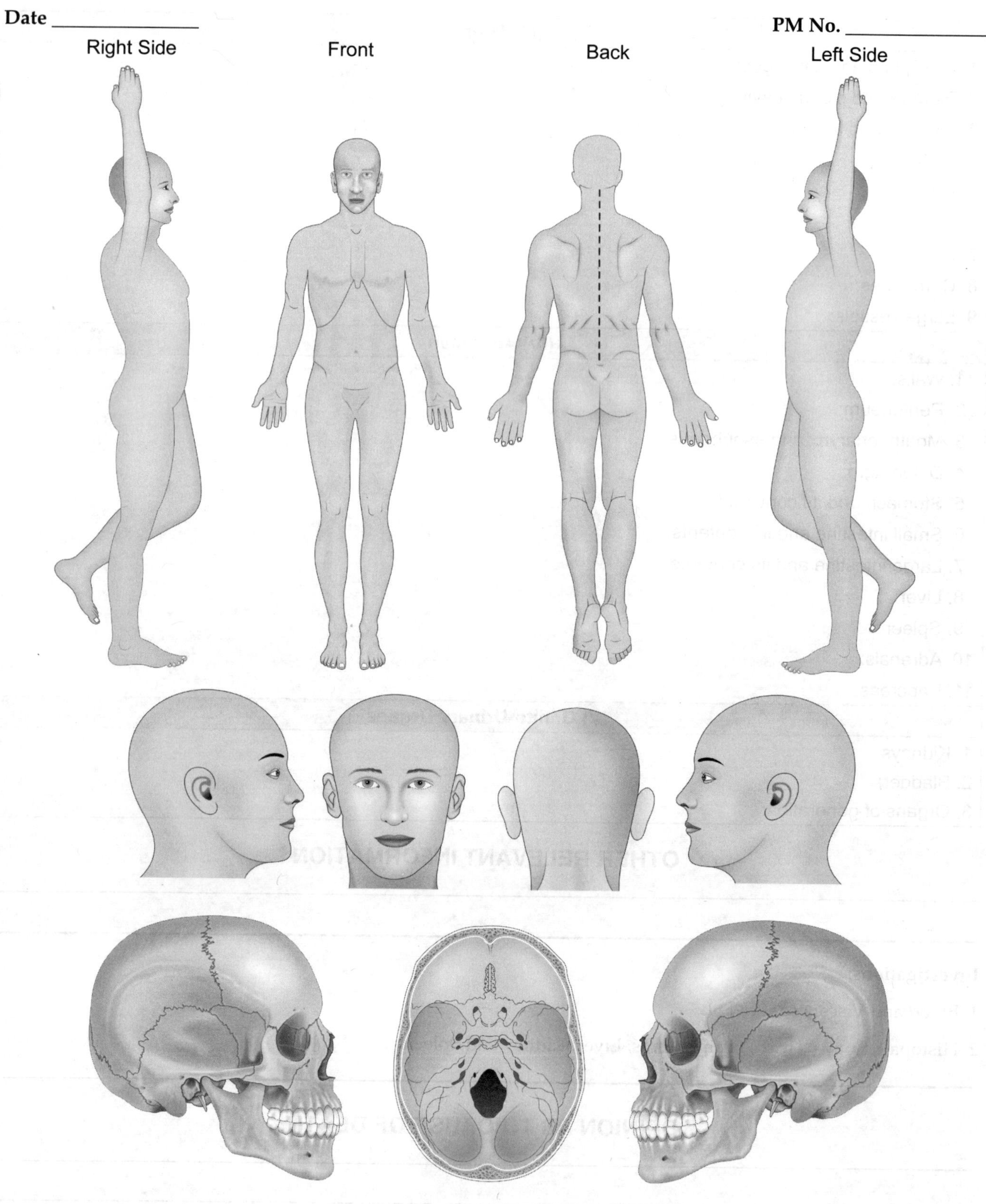

Signature of the Doctor
Name, Designation and Seal

EX. 6.4.15: POSTMORTEM REPORT

Department of Forensic Medicine

PM No.: ___________________

Dated: ___________________

Name of deceased ____

Father's Name/Husband's Name ____

Name ___________________ Sex ___________________ Religion ___________________ Cast ___________

Residence ____ P.O. ___________________________

Tehsil___________________________Thana___________________________Distt.___________________

Date & Time (Body brought for autopsy) ____

Body brought by   Body identified by

1.   1.

2.

3.   2.

4.

Police Post/Police Station

DATE AND HOUR OF

Death	PM Examination of Body	Dispatch of Matter to Chemical Examiner

Symptoms observed before death/information furnished by Police/Relative: ___________________________________

(I) External Appearance

1. Condition of subject body built, length, PM changes:

2. List of AM/PM wounds, type, position, size, mark of ligature/and other findings:

(II) Cranium and Spinal Cord
Note: The spinal canal need not be examined unless any indiction of injury exists.
1. Scalp, Skull and Vertebrae
2. Membranes
3. Brain
4. Spinal Cord

(III) Thorax
1. Walls, Ribs and Cartilages
2. Pleurae
3. Larynx and Trachea
4. Right Lung
5. Left Lung
6. Pericardium
7. Heart
8. Large Vessels
9. Right Coronary
10. Left Coronary

(IV) Abdomen
1. Walls
2. Peritoneum
3. Mouth, Pharynx and Esophagus
4. Stomach and its contents
5. Small intestines and its contents
6. Large intestines and its contents
7. Liver
8. Spleen
9. Kidneys
10. Bladder
11. Organs of generation: External and Internal

(V) Muscles, Bones and Joints			
Injury	Disease or Deformity	Fracture	Dislocation

(VI) Opinion of the Medical Officer

Probable time that elapsed—

(a) Between injury and death ____

(b) Between death and post-mortem ____

Abstract of chemical examinar's report, if any

List of wearing apparels:

1.   5.

2.   6.

3.   7.

4.

Body handover to police ____

Other articles handed over to police, if any ____

Viscera for FSL:

Jar I   Packet of preservative

Jar II

Vial I

Vial II   Sample Seal

Signature ________________

Name ________________

Designation ________________

Date ___________

PMR No. ___________

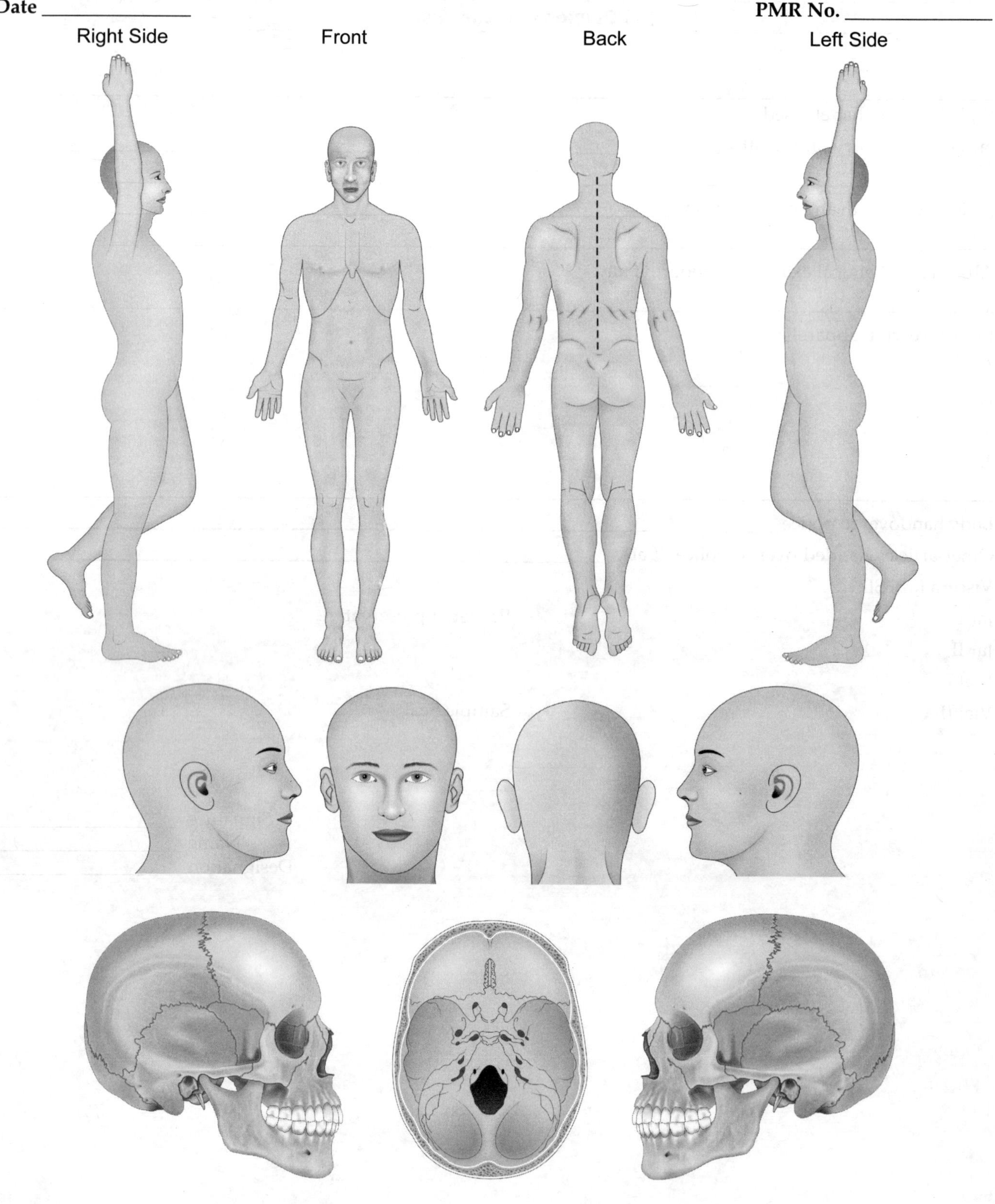

____
Signature of the Doctor
Name, Designation and Seal

LABELS TO BE ATTACHED TO MATERIAL SENT FOR CHEMICAL ANALYSIS

Department of Forensic Medicine and Toxicology

Viscera/Blood for Chemical Analysis

P.M. No. ________________   Date ______________

Bottle No. ____________

Name of the deceased ______________________________________ Age ___________ years Sex: _____________

Contents of this bottle: ____

Preservative: Saturated solution of sodium chloride/Sodium fluoride

Signature of the Medical Officer

Department of Forensic Medicine and Toxicology

Sample preservative

P.M. No. ______________   Date ______________

Bottle No. ____________

Name of the deceased ______________________________________ Age ___________ years Sex: _____________

Contents of this bottle: Saturated solution of sodium chloride/Sodium fluoride (preservative used)

Signature of the Medical Officer

LABEL TO BE AFFIXED ON THE SEALED BOX OF VISCERA

Department of Forensic Medicine and Toxicology

Materials: 1. Stomach, intestine and its contents, 2. Part of liver and half of each kidney, 3. Blood, 4. Urine, 5. Saturated solution of saline, 5. Sodium fluoride

P.M. No ______________   Date: ______________

Name of the deceased: ______________ Age ______________ years   Sex: _________________

FIR No. ________________ of ____ police station.

Place: ______________

Signature of the Medical Officer
Name, Designation and Seal

EX. 6.5: REPORT FORWARDED WITH THE VISCERA SENT FOR CHEMICAL ANALYSIS

Department of Forensic Medicine and Toxicology

____

To

The Chemical Examiner,

Govt. of _________________

______________________________ (District/City)

Subject: Viscera for chemical analysis for suspected ____ poisoning

Sir/Madam

I am forwarding the case particulars and below mentioned material through

Mr. ____ P.C. No _________________________________ for chemical analysis and certificate.

P.M. No. _________________________   Dated: _________________

Name of the deceased:_______________________________ Age _____________ years,   Sex __________________

FIR No. ____ of ____________________________________ police station.

Materials:

a.   A cloth covered sealed box with 10 seals containing:
1.   Stomach and part of intestine with its contents
2.   Part of liver and one half of each kidney
3.   Blood
4.   Urine
5.   Saturated saline (sample of preservative for 1 and 2)
6.   Sodium fluoride (sample of preservative for 3 and 4)

b.   A sealed envelope with 5 seals containing
1.   Request for chemical analysis
2.   Copy of PM report
3.   ____________ number of inquest papers duly signed
4.   Sample seal

Alleged cause of death as per inquest ____

Poisoning/drug suspected ____

Examination required: Quantitative and qualitative analysis for drugs/poisons suspected.

I request you that the report may be sent to the undersigned at the earliest.

Yours faithfully,

____

Place _________________   Signature of the Doctor

Date _________________   Name, Designation and Seal

EX. 6.6: REQUISITION FOR HISTOPATHOLOGICAL EXAMINATION

Department of Forensic Medicine and Toxicology

To

The Professor/Medical Officer I/C,

Department of Pathology

____

Subject: Histopathological examination of specimens preserved during the postmortem examination (Ref.: PM. No. ___________ dated _____________)

Sir/Madam,

I request that the histopathological examination of the following specimens, preserved from the dead body of

Mr/Ms ________________________________, S/D/W of _________________________________

aged _______________ years, involved in FIR No _________________of ______________ police station may be conducted, as the findings of such examination are absolutely necessary for furnishing opinion as to cause of death.

The alleged cause of death as per requisition for postmortem examination was _________________________________

____

Relevant findings at autopsy:

Organs/Specimens sent: *(Tick '✓')*

☐ Heart (whole, cut open)

☐ Brain (_________________________________)

☐ Lungs (_________________________________)

☐ Liver (_________________________________)

☐ Spleen (_________________________________)

☐ Kidneys (_________________________________)

☐ Pancreas (_________________________________)

☐ Female genitals (uterus, fallopian tubes, ovaries, vagina)

☐ Others (_________________________________)

I am sending the specimens in sealed packet and preserved in 10% formalin through H.C./P.C. No. _____________.
I request you that the results of histopathology report may be made ready at the earliest, so as to be collected through police.

With regards,

____

Signature of the Doctor

Place ___________

Name, Designation and Seal

Date ___________

EX. 6.7: FINAL OPINION AS TO CAUSE OF DEATH

Department of Forensic Medicine and Toxicology

____

To   Date _____________

The Investigating Officer,

______________________Police Station

______________________ (District/City)

Subject: Final opinion regarding PM report No. _______________ dated _______________

Ref:

a.   Chemical Examiner's report no. ___________________________________ dated _______________

b.   Histopathology report no. _______________________________ dated _______________

c.   Microbiology/Biochemistry report No. _____________________ dated ___________

As per requisition from the ____ of _________________________________

police station dated ____, postmortem examination was conducted on the body of

Mr/Ms ____ S/D/W of ____

aged about _____________________ years, involved in FIR No. _______________ of _______________ police

station and the P.M. report No. _______________ dated ___________ was issued by the undersigned.

The opinion as to cause of death was reserved pending results of chemical analysis of viscera and/or other material objects preserved from the body. (_Strike off if not applicable_).

The certificate of chemical analysis number _______________dated ___________of the above said viscera and other

materials were received by me on _________________.

Opinion

Based on the postmortem findings and results of laboratory examinations, I am of the opinion that the cause of death in above mentioned case was:

i.   Immediate cause ____

ii.   Due to ____

____

Signature of the Doctor

Place ___________   Name, Designation and Seal

Date ___________

____

Received final opinion of PM report No. _________________.

Name____P.C. No. _________________________P.S. _________________

____

Signature and Date

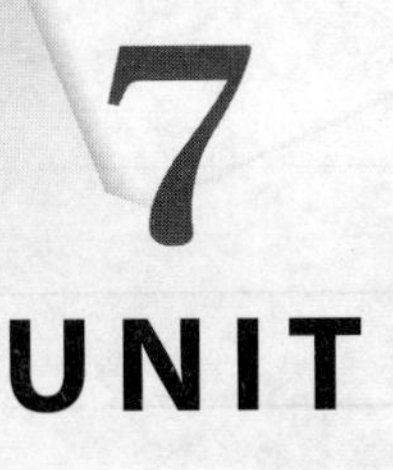

7 UNIT

Project

Case reports help students gain a deeper understanding of a topic—it serves as source of knowledge and important means for education and learning as he/she has to search and read extensively on that topic. They also act as an excellent introduction to academic writing. Doing a literature review, structuring a manuscript and learning how to revise the article are skills worth developing during their undergraduate days. The students will find abstract medical knowledge easier to remember when linked to a subject/patient. Case reports are generally related to unusual or previously unreported condition or findings. However, to keep it simple for the first time authors, this can be any case of that he/she has seen during the emergency or autopsy posting.

The student is required to workup and submit one case report within the stipulated deadline announced by the department. This case report may include any road traffic accident, burns, electrocution, firearm injury, sharp force injury, blunt force injury, fall from height, sexual offences, impotency, poisoning or any other medico-legal case that he/she has observed in the emergency. The autopsy case may include any accidental deaths, burns, hanging, strangulation, throttling, drowning, firearm deaths, sexual murder, fall from height, poisoning deaths, etc.

SCHEME OF WRITING THE REPORT

Important Considerations

1. *'De-identification' of the individual:* In order to maintain confidentiality, the patient's name, address and other identifiers such as hospital registration number must not be used. In photographs, masking (covering a subject's face or eyes) is done, and radiological images are anonymized to prevent identification.
2. *Obtain informed consent:* It is important to obtain written consent from the patient, if the student is taking any medico-legal case in the emergency. During the consent process, the student must explain the purpose of the study, and also take specific consent if he/she wish to include photographs.
3. *Data collection:* Before beginning to write the case itself, the student should gather all of the materials relevant to the case—clinical notes, laboratory reports, X-rays, photographs, etc.—and form a clear picture of the case that he/she wish to write. Once written, check the spelling and grammar.
4. *Literature review:* A literature review on a medical database such as PubMed, Med-Ind, Embase, Google Scholar or Medline can be used to check if there have been any similar cases. Previously published case reports will help improve understanding of the topic.

How to Write the Case Report

Case reports should encompass the following sections: title, abstract with keywords, introduction with a literature review, description of the case including a MLR or PMR, discussion that includes a detailed literature review and a conclusion (Checklist is given in **Table 7.1**).

Table 7.1: Checklist for writing case reports.

Title
• Should be brief and informative.
Abstract
• Word limit of 150–250 words.
• No abbreviations, no references.
Introduction
• Should be concise and attract the reader's attention.
• Similar cases that have been reported previously are described briefly.
Case report
• Describe the history of the incident.
• Provide details of the presentation and examination, including those from imaging and laboratory studies. Describe briefly the treatment and diagnosis.
• Provide details of the examination findings in postmortem report.
• Fill up the medico-legal report or postmortem report in proper format.
• Figures, illustrations, photographs, tables, X-rays, CT scans, etc.
• Informed consent form (in medico-legal reports).
Discussion
• Summarize the essential findings and compare the case report with the literature.
• Literature should be relevant to the topic.
Conclusion
• State the lessons that may be learnt from the case report.
References
• Limited to 15–20 recent ones in Vancouver style.

Title

The first page of the project should be dedicated to the title page. The 'title' should be a clear and short description of the case along with student's full name, batch, roll no., institutional address and e-mail address. Abbreviations within the title should be avoided.

Abstract

It is better to write the abstract, once the main body of text has been completed. Abstracts should be concise, about 150–250 words. It summaries the case and gives an overall idea about the content of the case report. Abbreviations or references within the abstract should not be used.

Students can write the abstracts using one of two styles, *unstructured* (narrative) or *structured*. A narrative abstract consists of a short version of the whole paper. There are no headings within the narrative abstract. A structured abstract uses subheadings, and can be divided into three sections: (1) Background: an introduction about this case; (2) Case presentation: brief details of the case (brief history and findings); and (3) Conclusions: brief conclusion of what the reader should learn from the case report.

Keywords

Provide 2–5 keywords which will be used when searching for the case report using a search engine.

Introduction

Briefly summarize the background and context of this case report. This should be from the standpoint of those without specialist knowledge in the area, explaining the background of the topic. If similar cases have been reported previously, describe them briefly. A more detailed literature review is done in the discussion. Each time, when referred to a previous study, cite the reference (usually at the end of the sentence, in superscripts).

Case Description

Write in a narrative style, restricting to the relevant information. The case report is best presented in chronological order, typically comprising of patient's demographic information (without any details that could lead to the identification of the patient), history of the incident, any relevant medical or past history of the patient, examination findings, starting with the vital signs presented at the examination, investigative results, including imaging and laboratory results, brief management and diagnosis.

All important negative findings should also be provided. Include two or three photographs to keep the reader engaged. Photographs should be of good quality along with scale and date. In the case of surgery and pathology consults, a comprehensive summary of the surgical procedure and detailed pathologist's report should be included. X-rays or other images are included, if they are clear enough to be easily reproduced.

- *Management and outcome:* Briefly describe the plan for care, as well as the care which was actually provided and the outcome.
- The medico-legal report or the postmortem report in proper format should be included in the report.
- Final opinion in medico-legal reports should be based on the diagnostic results (testing, imaging) and specialists' opinions (pathological reports, surgical reports, etc.) which should be given at the end of case description.

Discussion

The discussion is the most important section of the case report. It evaluates the case and compare and contrast with the published literature. Start by briefly expanding on introduction, then sum up the current literature related to the case. Describe what has already been reported about this topic, what are the main findings, explain those findings and how the present case differs or conforms to those previously published literature.

Give information about the condition in question, such as the definitions, basic epidemiology, pathophysiology, clinical presentation and investigations.

Further Research/Suggestions

The student may give his/her suggestions for further research. Lessons learnt from the case with justifiable evidence-based recommendations may be included.

Conclusion

State clearly the main conclusions of the case report and give a clear explanation of its importance and relevance.

Acknowledgments

Students should acknowledge anyone who contributed towards the article by making substantial contributions or who was involved in drafting the manuscript.

References

Students must search for and cite published case reports that are relevant to the case. References should be listed in the Vancouver or Harvard style. There should be not more than 15–20 current references (within the last 5 years, unless it is of historic interest). The Vancouver system of referencing is cited below:

Books

1. Author Surname Initials. Title: subtitle. Edition (if not the first). Place of publication: Publisher; Year.
   a. Mason J. Concepts in dental public health. Philadelphia: Lippincott Williams and Wilkins; 2005.
   b. Dionne RA, Phero JC, Becker DE (eds). Management of pain and anxiety in the dental office. Philadelphia: WB Saunders; 2002.
   c. Fauci AS, Braunwald E, Kasper DL, Hauser SL, Longo DL, Jameson JL, et al. (eds). Harrison's principles of internal medicine. 17th ed. New York: McGraw Hill; 2008. (if more than 6 authors/editors)

Chapter in a Book

Alexander RG. Considerations in creating a beautiful smile. In: Romano R (ed). The art of the smile. London: Quintessence Publishing; 2005. p. 187-210.

E-book

Irfan A. Protocols for predictable aesthetic dental restorations [Internet]. Oxford: Blackwell Munksgaard; 2006 [cited 2009 May 21]. Available from Netlibrary: http://cclsw2.vcc.ca:2048/login?url=http://www.netLibrary.com/urlapi.asp?action=summary&v=1&bookid=181691.

Organization as Author

Canadian Dental Hygienists Association. Dental hygiene: definition and scope. Ottawa: Canadian Dental Hygienists Association; 1995.

No Author/Editor

Scott's Canadian dental directory 2008. 9th ed. Toronto: Scott's Directories; 2007.

Government Document

Canada. Environmental Health Directorate. Radiation protection in dentistry: recommended safety procedures for the use of dental X-ray equipment. Safety Code 30. Ottawa: Ministry of Health; 2000.

Format for Journal Articles

Author Surname Initials. Title of article. Title of journal, abbreviated. Date of Publication: Volume Number (Issue Number): Page Numbers.

Haas AN, de Castro GD, Moreno T, Susin C, Albandar JM, Oppermann RV, et al. Azithromycin as a adjunctive treatment of aggressive periodontitis: 12-months randomized clinical trial. J Clin Periodontol. 2008; 35(8): 696-704.

Journal Article from a Website

Tasdemir T, Yesilyurt C, Ceyhanli KT, Celik D, Er K. Evaluation of apical filling after root canal filling by 2 different techniques. J Can Dent Assoc [Internet]. 2009 [cited 2009 Jun 14];75(3):[about 5pp.]. Available from: http://www.cda-adc.ca/jcda/vol-75/issue-3/201.html.

Dictionary, Encyclopedia or Similar Reference Book

Unsigned

Mosby's dental dictionary. 2nd ed. St. Louis: Mosby Elsevier; 2008. Frenotomy; p. 273.

Signed (and Online)

Murchison DF. Dental emergencies. In: Merck Manual of Diagnosis and Therapy [Internet]. 18th ed. Whitehouse Station (NJ): Merck; 2009 [last modified 2009 Mar; cited 2009 Jun 23]. Available from: http://www.merck.com/mmpe/sec08/ch096/ch096a.html?qt=dental&alt=sh.

Newspaper Articles

1. Fayerman P. Women must now wait to 40 for publicly paid amnio test. Vancouver Sun. 2009 Jun 9; Sect. A: 5.
2. Health Canada issues warning over fake toothbrushes. The Globe and Mail [Internet]. 2009 April 10 [cited 2009 Jun 23]. Available from: http://www.theglobeandmail.com/news/national/health-canada-issues-warning-over-fake-toothbrushes/article973190/

Identification of Injuries, Poisons and Histopathological Slides

FM 14.9: Demonstrate ability to identify and prepare medico-legal inference from specimens obtained from various types of injuries e.g., abrasion, contusion, laceration, firearm wounds, burns, head injury and fracture of bone.

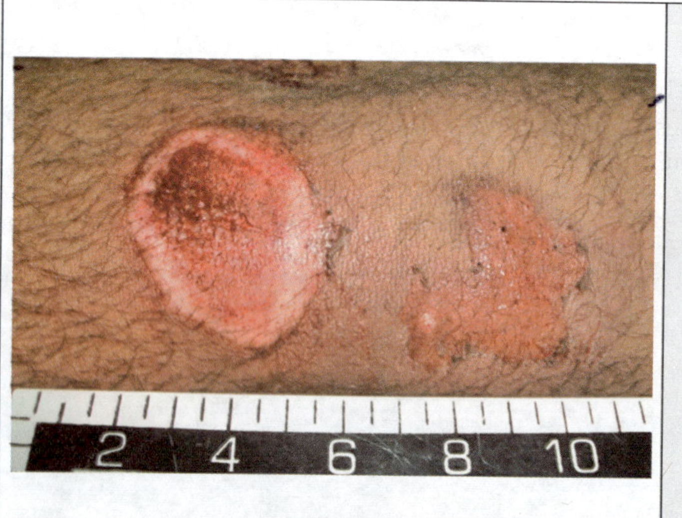

Identify the type of wound:

Force/weapon used:

Time since injury:

Medico-legal inference:

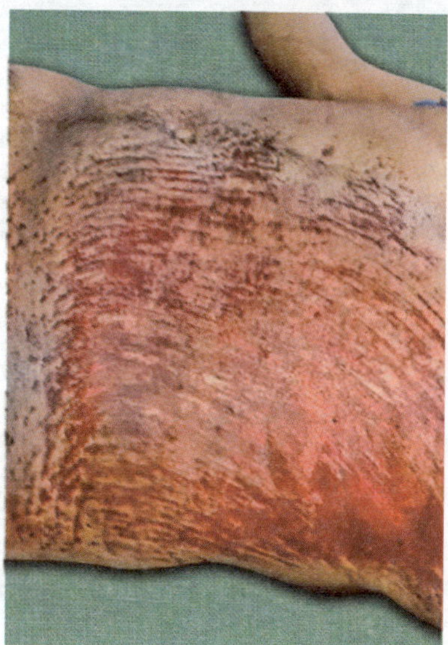

Identify the type of wound:

Force/weapon used:

Time since injury:

Medico-legal inference:

EX. 8.1B: IDENTIFICATION OF INJURIES

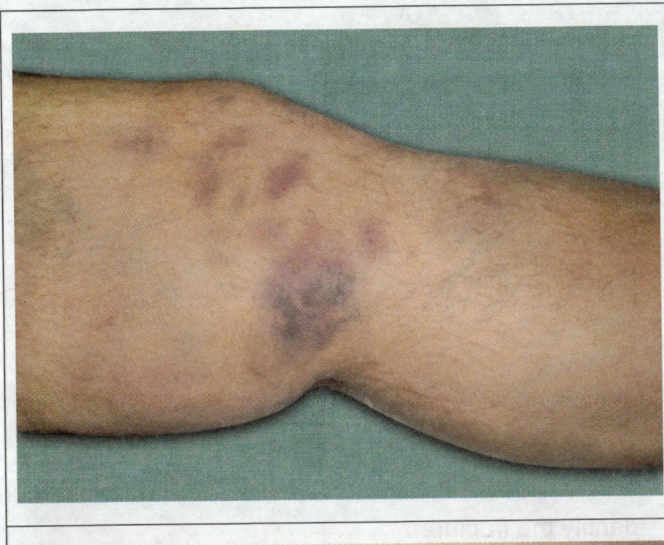

Identify the type of wound:

Force/weapon used:

Time since injury:

Medico-legal inference:

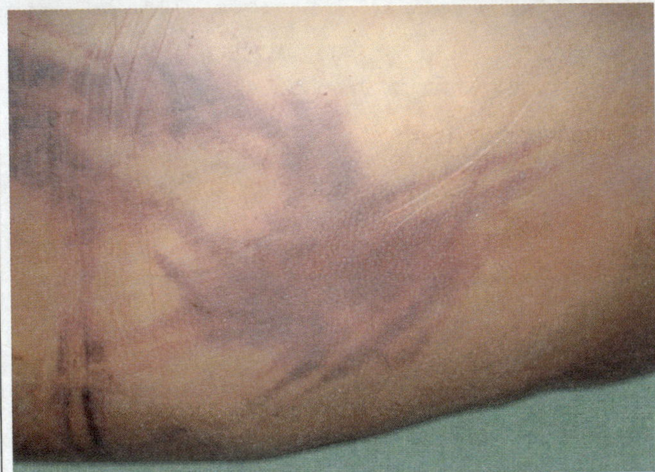

Identify the type of wound:

Force/weapon used:

Time since injury:

Medico-legal inference:

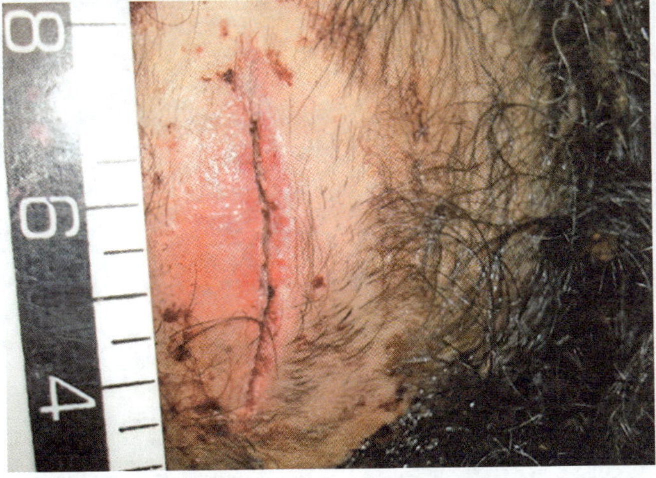

Identify the type of wound:

Force/weapon used:

Time since injury:

Medico-legal inference:

EX. 8.1C: IDENTIFICATION OF INJURIES

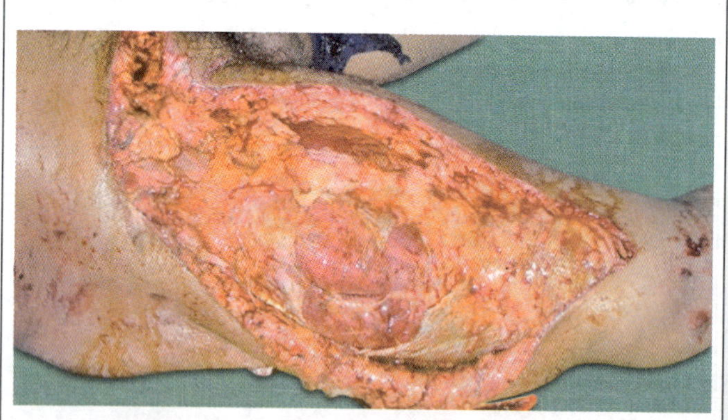

Identify the type of wound:

Force/weapon used:

Time since injury:

Medico-legal inference:

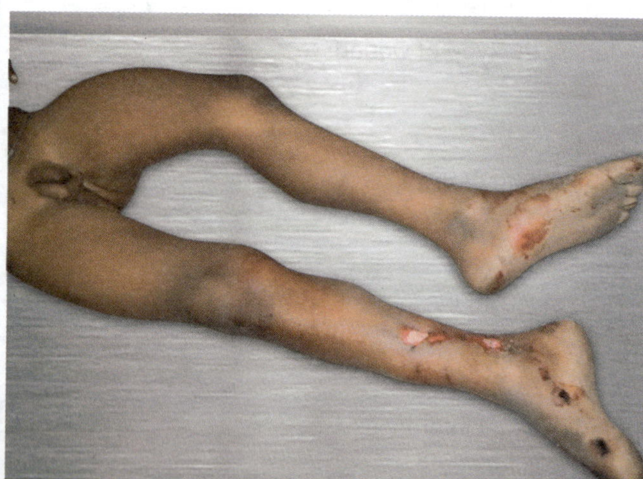

Identify the fracture:

Force/weapon used:

Medico-legal inference:

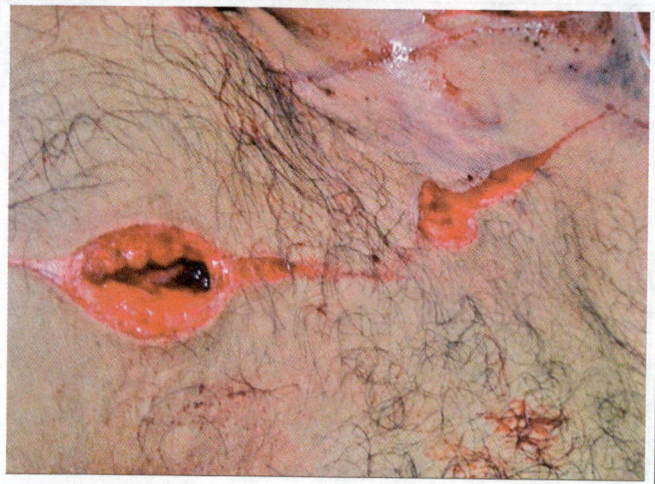

Identify the type of wound:

Force/weapon used:

Time since injury:

Medico-legal inference:

EX. 8.1D: IDENTIFICATION OF INJURIES

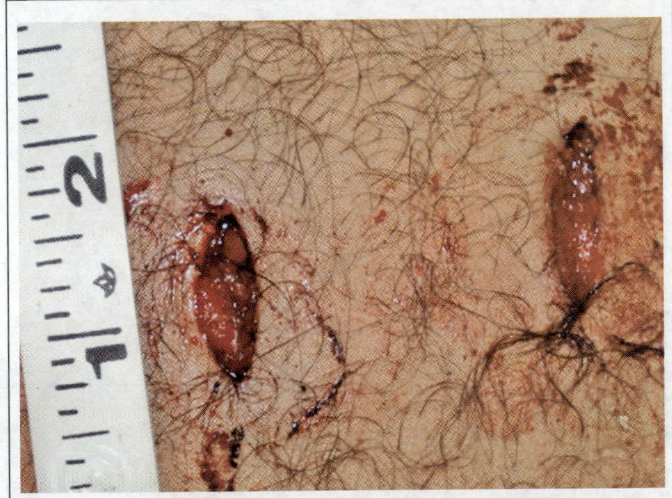

Identify the type of wound:

Force/weapon used:

Time since injury:

Medico-legal inference:

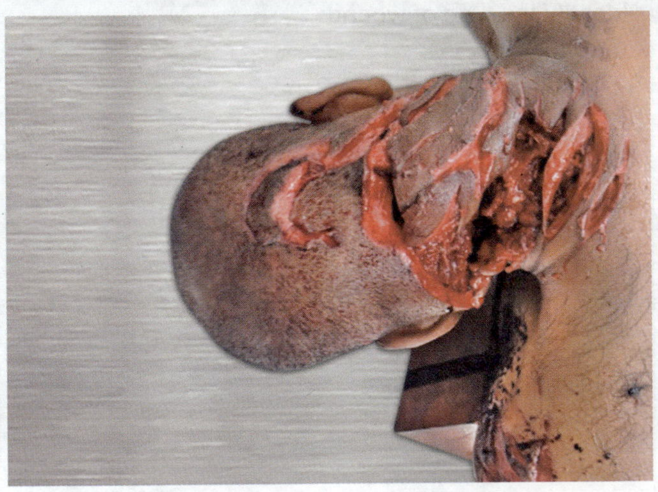

Identify the type of wound:

Force/weapon used:

Time since injury:

Medico-legal inference:

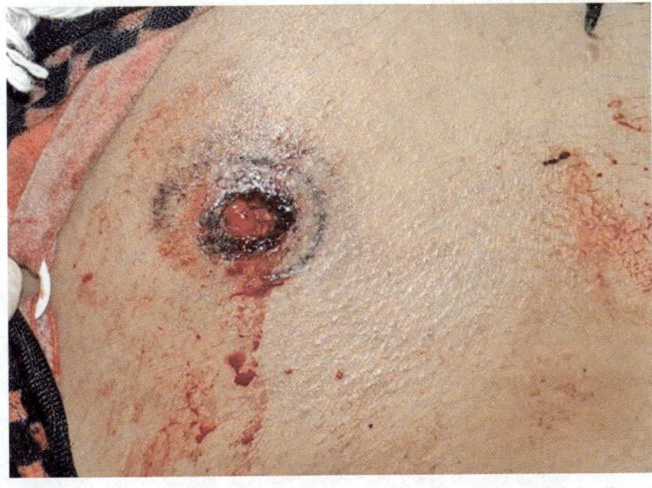

Identify the type of wound:

Force/weapon used:

Time since injury:

Medico-legal inference:

EX. 8.1E: IDENTIFICATION OF INJURIES

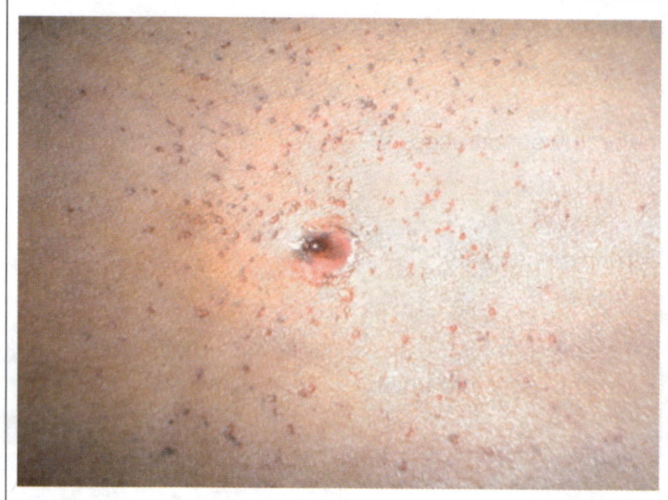

Identify the type of wound:

Force/weapon used:

Time since injury:

Medico-legal inference:

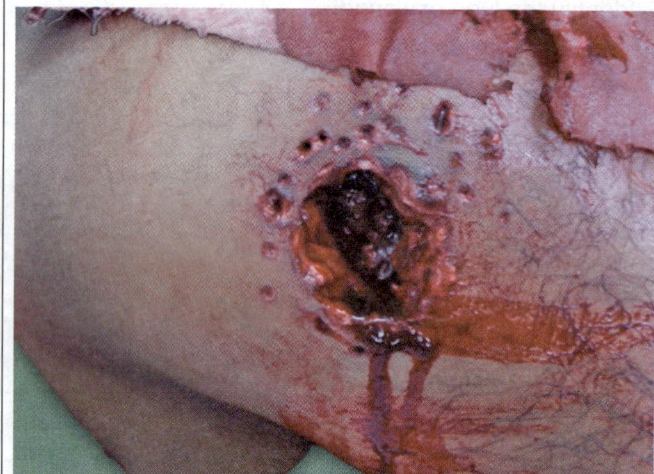

Identify the type of wound:

Force/weapon used:

Time since injury:

Medico-legal inference:

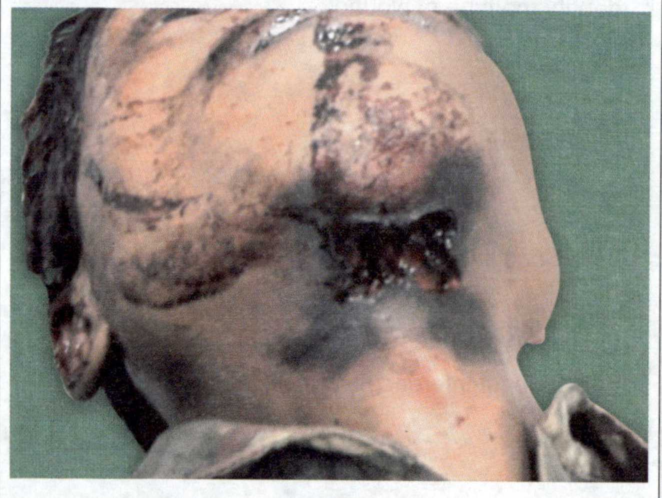

Identify the type of wound:

Force/weapon used:

Time since injury:

Medico-legal inference:

EX. 8.1F: IDENTIFICATION OF INJURIES

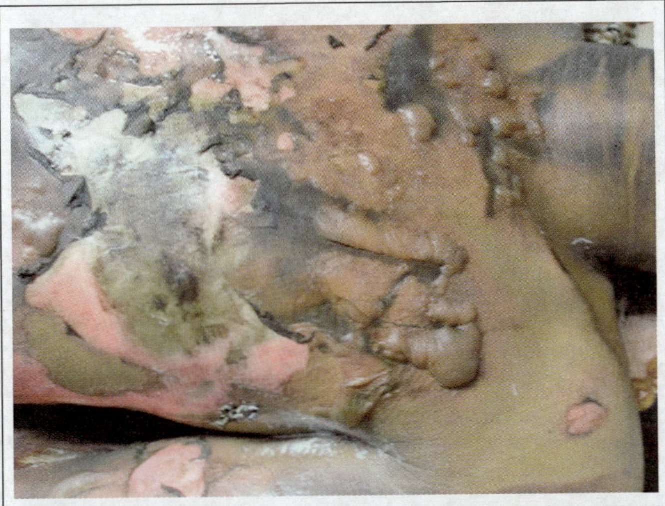

Identify the injury:

Causative agent and degree:

Medico-legal inference:

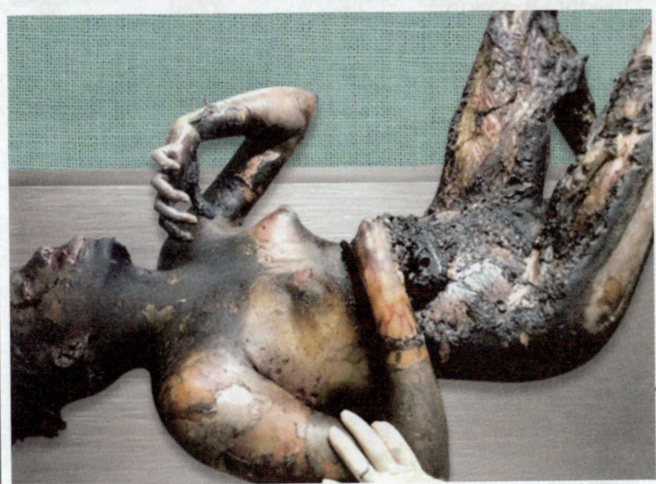

Identify the injury:

Causative agent and degree:

Medico-legal inference:

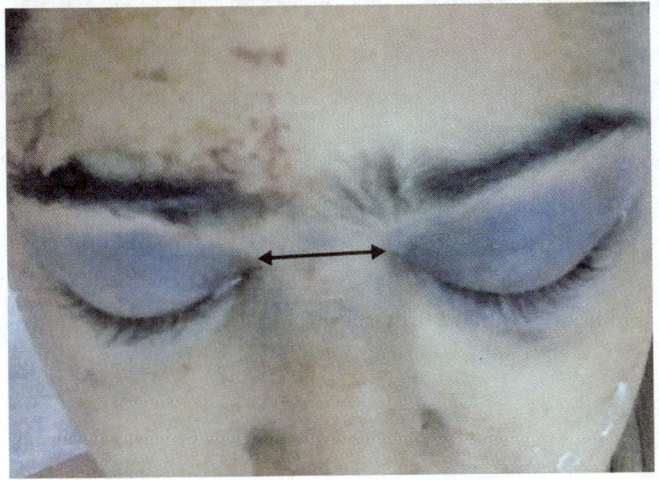

Identify the sign:

Cause:

Medico-legal inference:

EX. 8.1G: IDENTIFICATION OF INJURIES

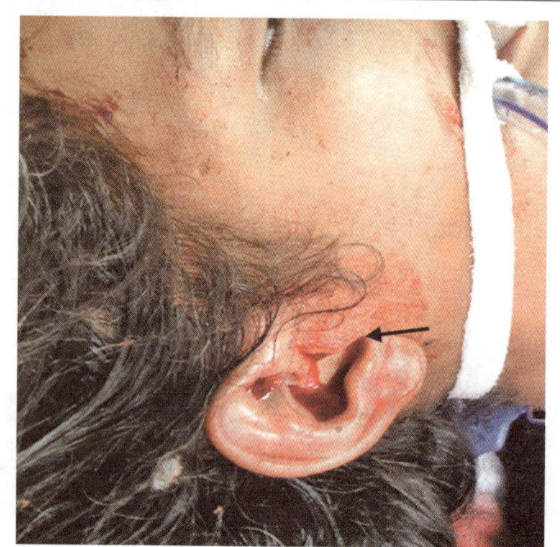

Identify the sign/injury:

Cause:

Medico-legal inference:

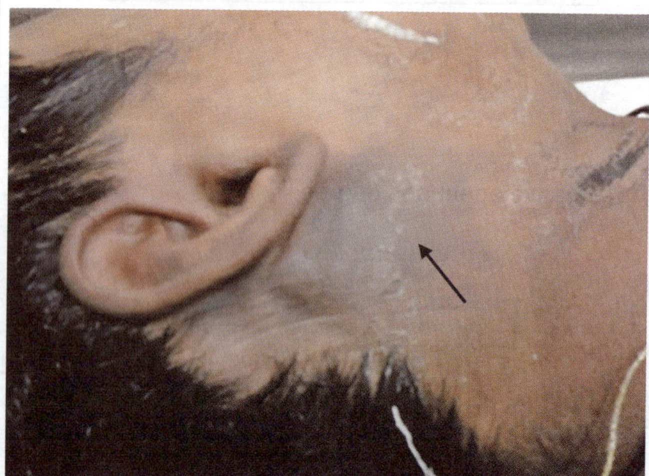

Identify the sign:

Cause:

Medico-legal inference:

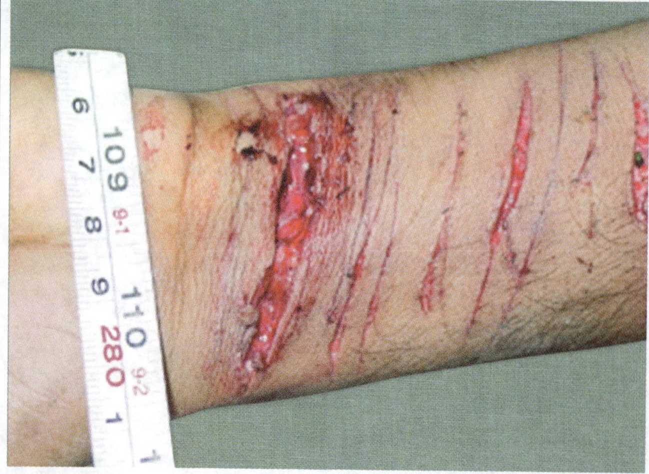

Identify the injury:

Cause:

Medico-legal inference:

EX. 8.1H: IDENTIFICATION OF INJURIES

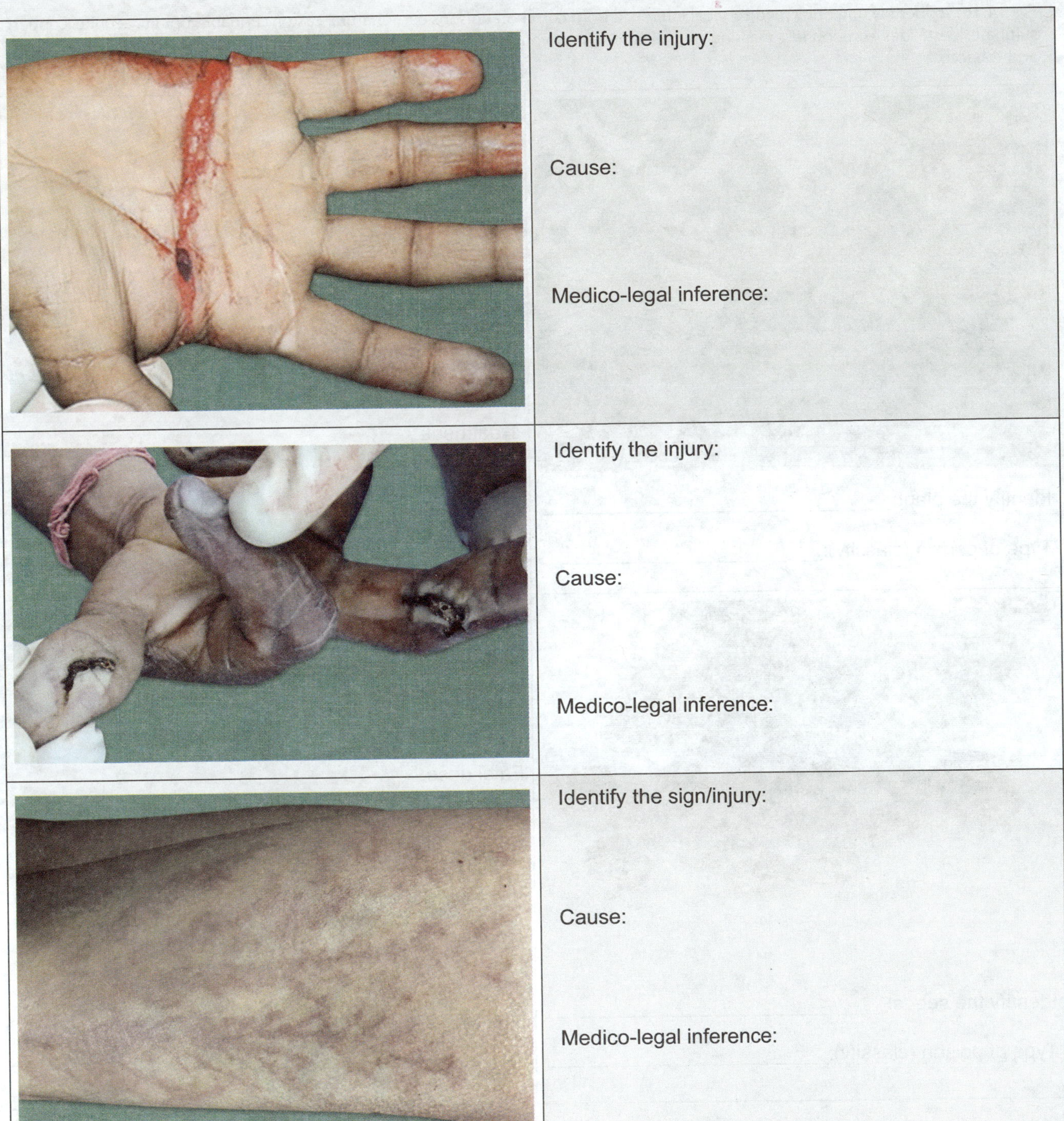

Identify the injury:

Cause:

Medico-legal inference:

Identify the injury:

Cause:

Medico-legal inference:

Identify the sign/injury:

Cause:

Medico-legal inference:

EX. 8.2A: IDENTIFICATION OF COMMON POISONS

FM 14.16: To identify and draw medico-legal inference from common poisons e.g., dhatura, castor, cannabis, opium, aconite, copper sulphate, pesticides compounds, marking nut, oleander, nux vomica, abrus seeds, snakes, capsicum, calotropis, lead compounds and tobacco.

Characteristic features:

Active principles:

Fatal dose:

Signs and symptoms:

Treatment:

Identify the plant:_______________________________

Medico-legal inference:

Type of poison (classify):_________________________

Characteristic features:

Active principles:

Fatal dose:

Signs and symptoms:

Treatment:

Identify the seeds: _______________________________

Medico-legal inference:

Type of poison (classify):_________________________

EX. 8.2B: IDENTIFICATION OF COMMON POISONS

Identify the seeds: _______________________________

Type of poison (classify): _______________________

Characteristic features:

Active principles:

Fatal dose:

Signs and symptoms:

Treatment:

Medico-legal inference:

Identify the leaves: _______________________________

Type of poison (classify): _______________________

Characteristic features:

Active principles:

Various preparations:

Fatal dose:

Signs and symptoms:

Treatment:

Medico-legal inference:

EX. 8.2C: IDENTIFICATION OF COMMON POISONS

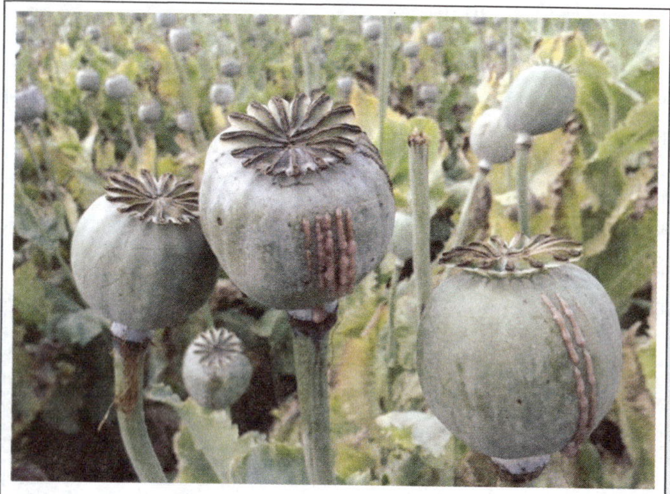

Identify the plant:_______________________________

Type of poison (classify):_______________________

Characteristic features:

Active principles:

Fatal dose:

Signs and symptoms:

Treatment:

Medico-legal inference:

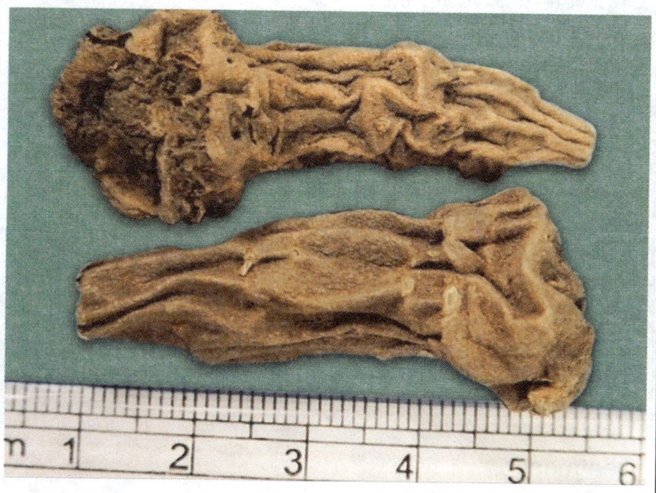

Identify the root:_______________________________

Type of poison (classify):_______________________

Characteristic features:

Active principles:

Fatal dose:

Signs and symptoms:

Treatment:

Medico-legal inference:

EX. 8.2D: IDENTIFICATION OF COMMON POISONS

Identify the poison:______________________________

Type of poison (classify):______________________

Characteristic features:

Fatal dose:

Signs and symptoms:

Treatment:

Medico-legal inference:

Identify the snake:______________________________

Type of poison (classify):______________________

Characteristic features:

Type of venom:

Fatal dose:

Signs and symptoms:

Treatment:

Medico-legal inference:

EX. 8.2E: IDENTIFICATION OF COMMON POISONS

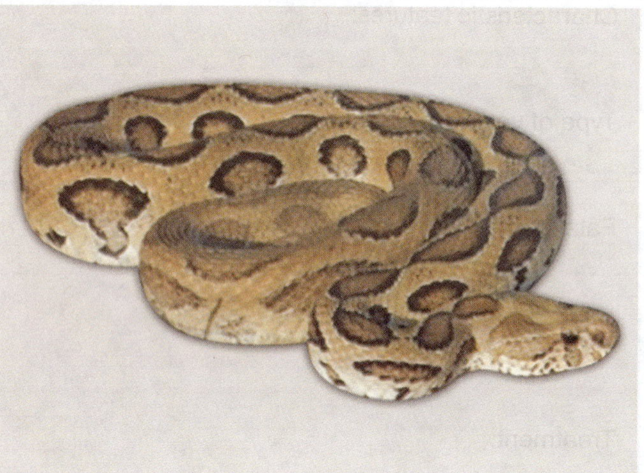

Identify the snake:________________________________

Type of poison (classify):___________________________

Characteristic features:

Type of venom:

Fatal dose:

Signs and symptoms:

Treatment:

Medico-legal inference:

Identify the snake:________________________________

Type of poison (classify):___________________________

Characteristic features:

Type of venom:

Fatal dose:

Signs and symptoms:

Treatment:

Medico-legal inference:

EX. 8.2F: IDENTIFICATION OF COMMON POISONS

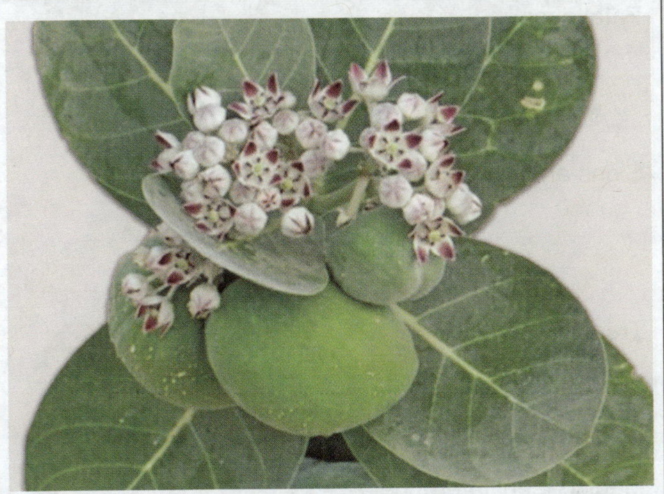

Identify the plant and the fruit:_____________________

Type of poison (classify):_____________________

Active principles:

Fatal dose:

Signs and symptoms:

Treatment:

Medico-legal inference:

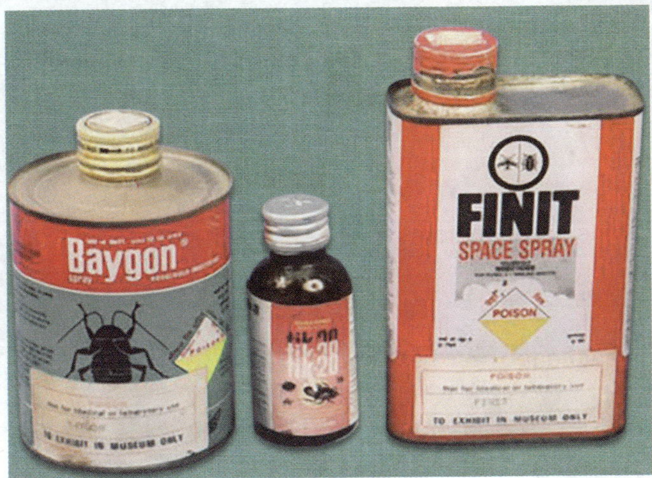

Identify the pesticide:_____________________

Type of poison (classify):_____________________

Fatal dose:

Signs and symptoms:

Treatment:

Medico-legal inference:

EX. 8.2G: IDENTIFICATION OF COMMON POISONS

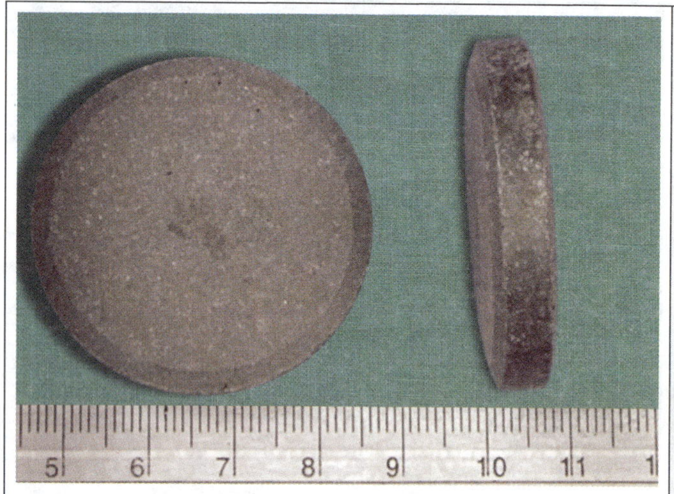

Identify the pesticide:______________________________

Type of poison (classify):______________________________

Fatal dose:

Signs and symptoms:

Treatment:

Medico-legal inference:

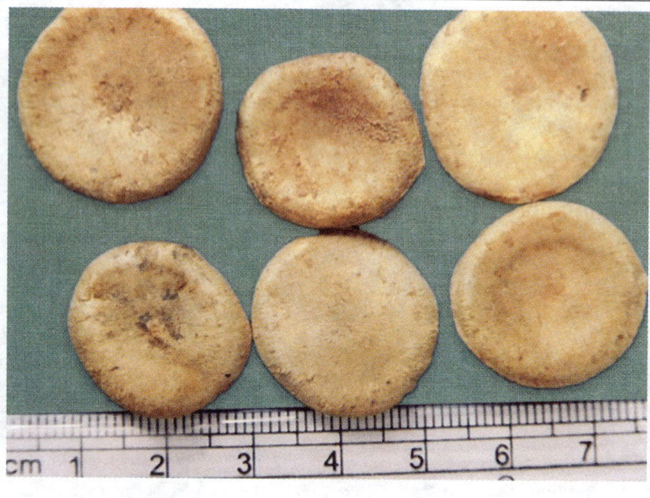

Identify the seeds:______________________________

Type of poison (classify):______________________________

Active principles:

Fatal dose:

Signs and symptoms:

Treatment:

Medico-legal inference:

EX. 8.2H: IDENTIFICATION OF COMMON POISONS

Identify the seeds:_______________________

Type of poison (classify):_______________________

Active principles:

Fatal dose:

Signs and symptoms:

Treatment:

Medico-legal inference:

Identify the seeds:_______________________

Type of poison (classify):_______________________

Active principles:

Fatal dose:

Signs and symptoms:

Treatment:

Medico-legal inference:

EX. 8.2I: IDENTIFICATION OF COMMON POISONS

Active component:

Fatal dose:

Signs and symptoms:

Treatment:

Medico-legal inference:

Identify the leaves:_______________________________

Type of poison (classify):_______________________________

Fatal dose:

Signs and symptoms:

Treatment:

Medico-legal inference:

Identify the poison:_______________________________

Type of poison (classify):_______________________________

EX. 8.3A: IDENTIFICATION OF HISTOPATHOLOGICAL SLIDES

To identify and prepare medico-legal inference from histopathological slides of myocardial infarction, tuberculosis, brain infarct, liver cirrhosis, brain hemorrhage, bone fracture, pulmonary edema, brain edema, soot particles, diatoms, wound healing and bronchopneumonia.

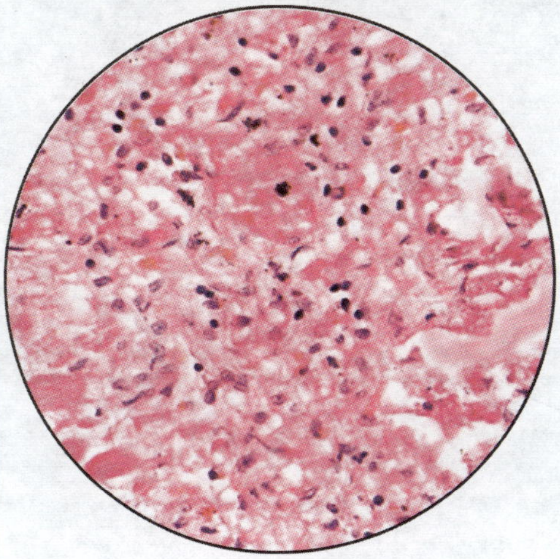

Draw a well labeled diagram of the slide *Myocardial infarction* shown above:

Findings: ____

____

Medico-legal inference: ____

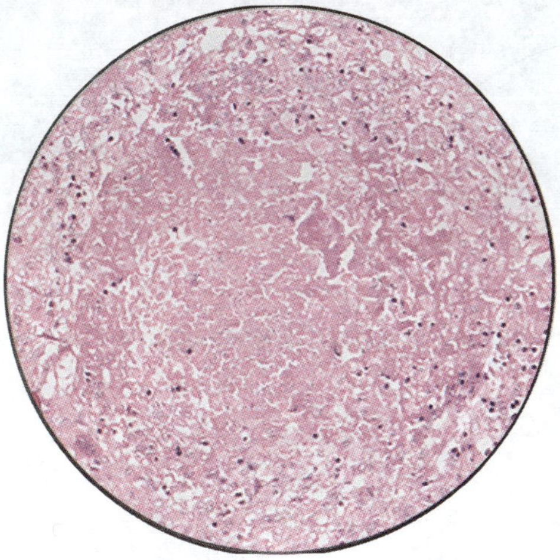

____

Draw a well labeled diagram of the slide *Tuberculosis of Lung* shown above:

Findings: ____

____

Medico-legal inference: ____

____

EX. 8.3B: IDENTIFICATION OF HISTOPATHOLOGICAL SLIDES

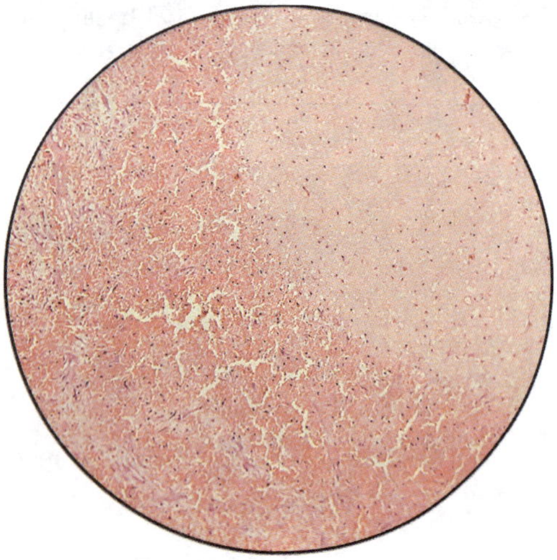

Draw a well labeled diagram of the slide *Brain infarct* shown above:

Findings: ____

____

Medico-legal inference: ____

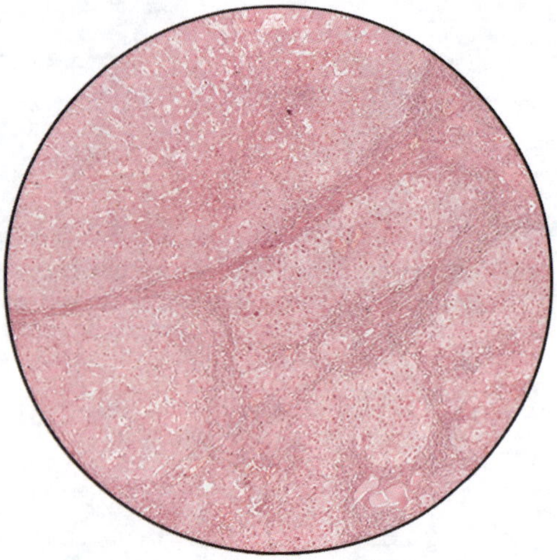

____

Draw a well labeled diagram of the slide *Liver cirrhosis* shown above:

Findings: ____

____

Medico-legal inference: ____

____

EX. 8.3C: IDENTIFICATION OF HISTOPATHOLOGICAL SLIDES

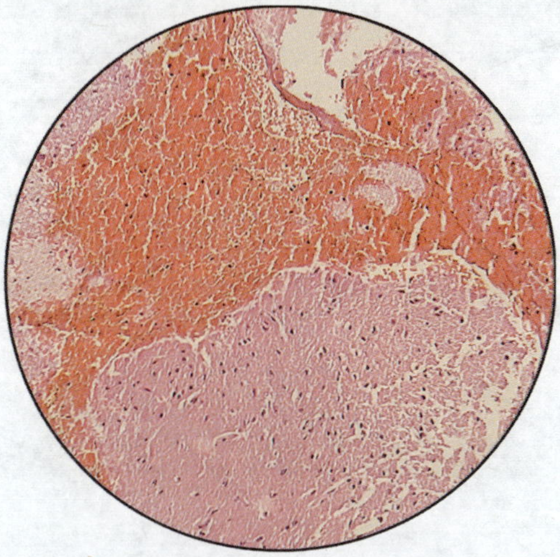

Draw a well labeled diagram of the slide *Brain hemorrhage* shown above:

Findings: ____

____

Medico-legal inference: ____

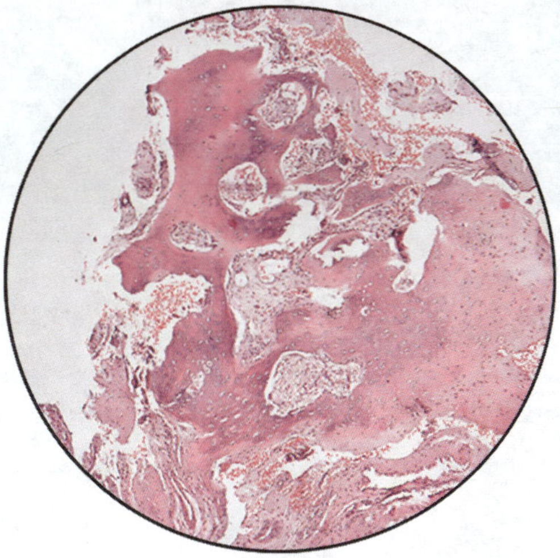

____

Draw a well labeled diagram of the slide *Bone fracture* shown above:

Findings: ____

____

Medico-legal inference: ____

____

EX. 8.3D: IDENTIFICATION OF HISTOPATHOLOGICAL SLIDES

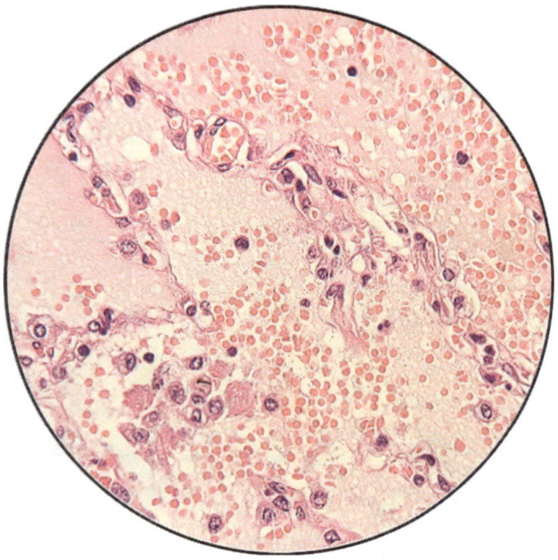

Draw a well labeled diagram of the slide *Pulmonary edema* shown above:

Findings: ____

____

Medico-legal inference: ____

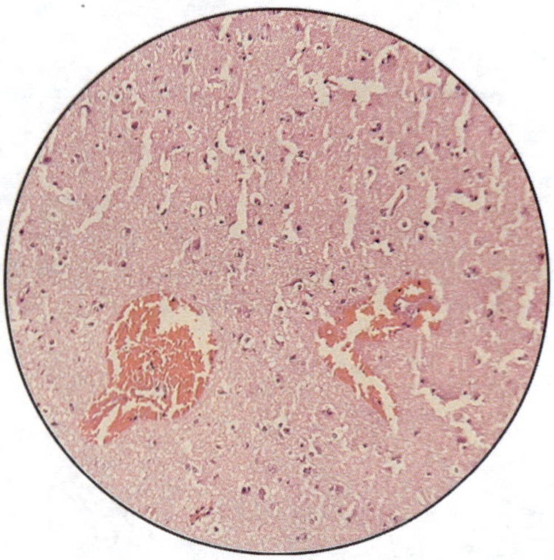

____

Draw a well labeled diagram of the slide *Brain edema* shown above:

Findings: ____

____

Medico-legal inference: ____

____

EX. 8.3E: IDENTIFICATION OF HISTOPATHOLOGICAL SLIDES

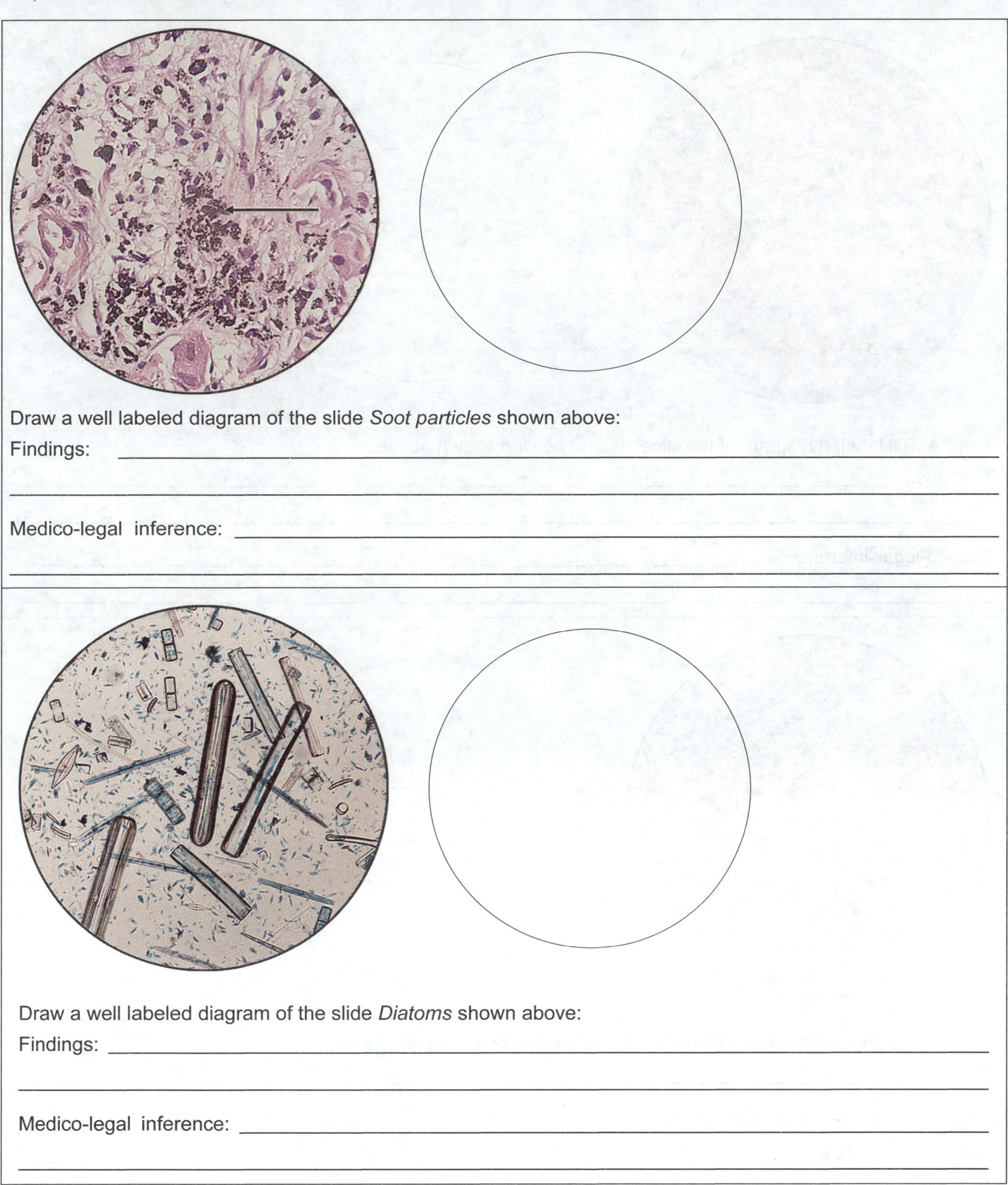

Draw a well labeled diagram of the slide *Soot particles* shown above:

Findings: ____

____

Medico-legal inference: ____

____

Draw a well labeled diagram of the slide *Diatoms* shown above:

Findings: ____

____

Medico-legal inference: ____

____

EX. 8.3F: IDENTIFICATION OF HISTOPATHOLOGICAL SLIDES

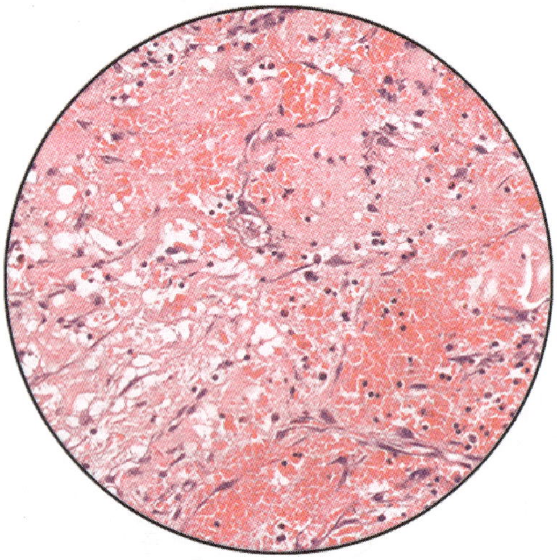

Draw a well labeled diagram of the slide *Wound healing* shown above:

Findings: ____

____

Medico-legal inference: ____

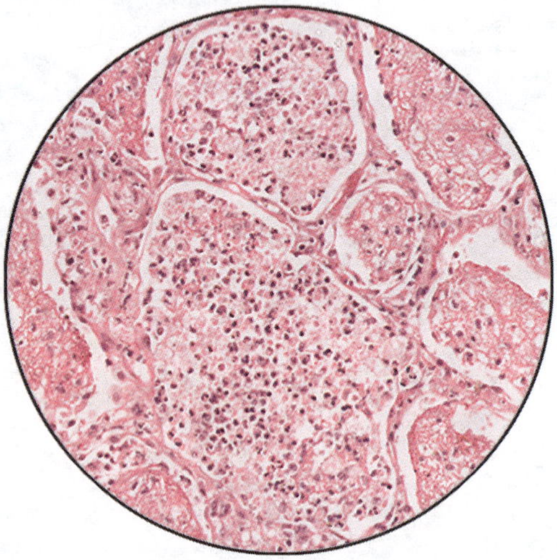

____

Draw a well labeled diagram of the slide *Bronchopneumonia* shown above:

Findings: ____

____

Medico-legal inference: ____

____

Self-Directed Learning (SDL)

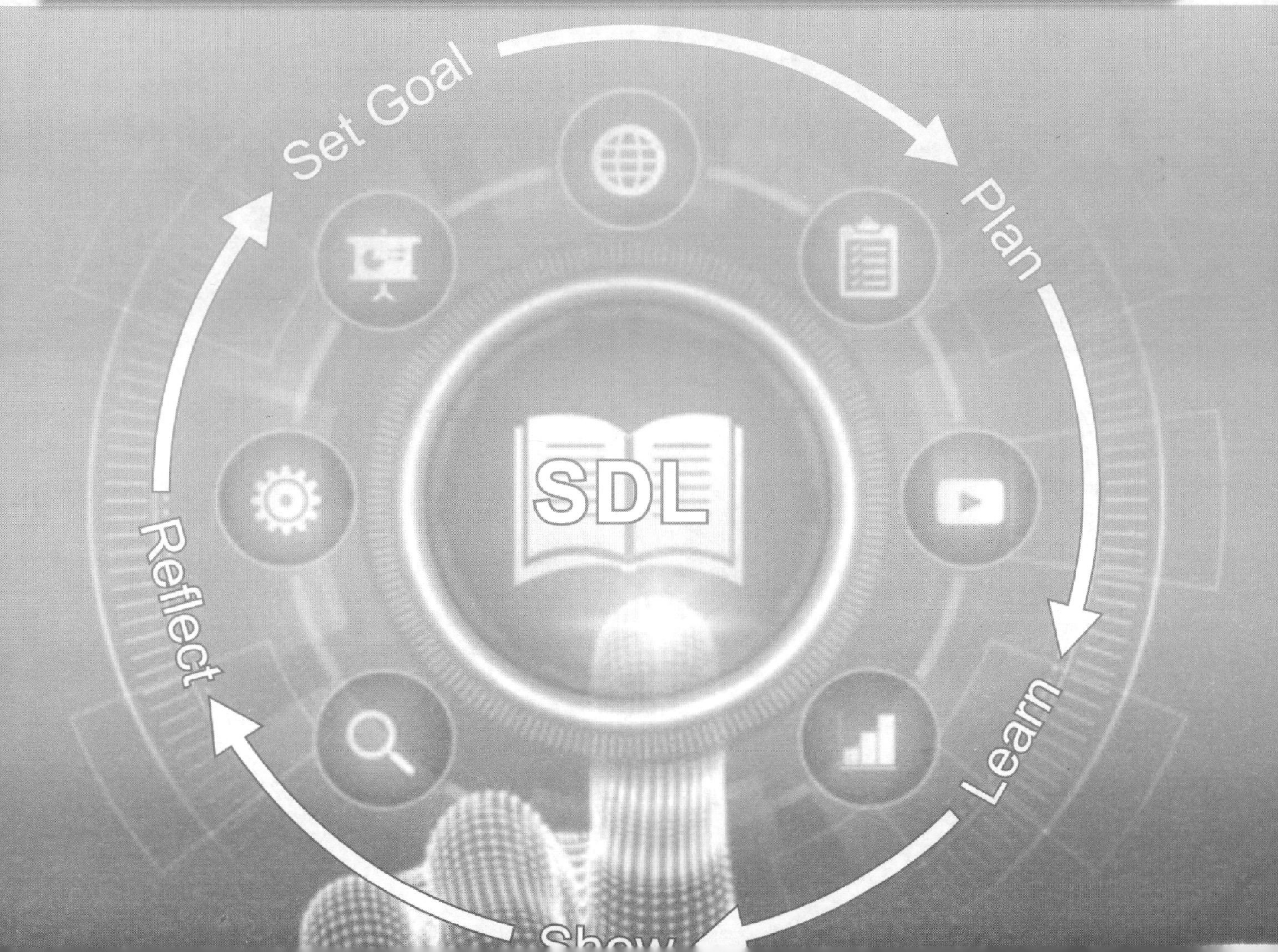

Self-Directed Learning (SDL)

SELF-DIRECTED LEARNING

Sl. No.	Date	Topic learnt	Mode of learning (quiz/seminar/any other mode)	Signature of teacher

Note: Total allotted SDL hours for Forensic Medicine and Toxicology in Second and Final Part (1) Professional MBBS is 10 hours.

SDL 1: REFLECTION ON SELF-DIRECTED LEARNING

Topic: ....

What happened:

....

....

....

....

....

....

So what:

....

....

....

....

....

....

....

What next:

....

....

....

....

....

....

Date   **Signature of Teacher-in-Charge**

SDL 2: REFLECTION ON SELF-DIRECTED LEARNING

Topic: ....

What happened:

....
....
....
....
....
....
....

So what:

....
....
....
....
....
....

What next:

....
....
....
....
....
....

Date   **Signature of Teacher-in-Charge**

SDL 3: REFLECTION ON SELF-DIRECTED LEARNING

Topic: ....

What happened:

....

....

....

....

....

....

So what:

....

....

....

....

....

....

What next:

....

....

....

....

....

Date   **Signature of Teacher-in-Charge**

SDL 4: REFLECTION ON SELF-DIRECTED LEARNING

Topic: ....

What happened:

....

....

....

....

....

....

....

So what:

....

....

....

....

....

....

What next:

....

....

....

....

....

....

Date   **Signature of Teacher-in-Charge**

SDL 5: REFLECTION ON SELF-DIRECTED LEARNING

Topic: ....

What happened:

....

....

....

....

....

....

So what:

....

....

....

....

....

....

....

What next:

....

....

....

....

....

Date   **Signature of Teacher-in-Charge**

SDL 6: REFLECTION ON SELF-DIRECTED LEARNING

Topic: ....

What happened:

....

....

....

....

....

....

So what:

....

....

....

....

....

....

What next:

....

....

....

....

....

Date   **Signature of Teacher-in-Charge**

3

Attitude, Ethics and Communication (AETCOM)

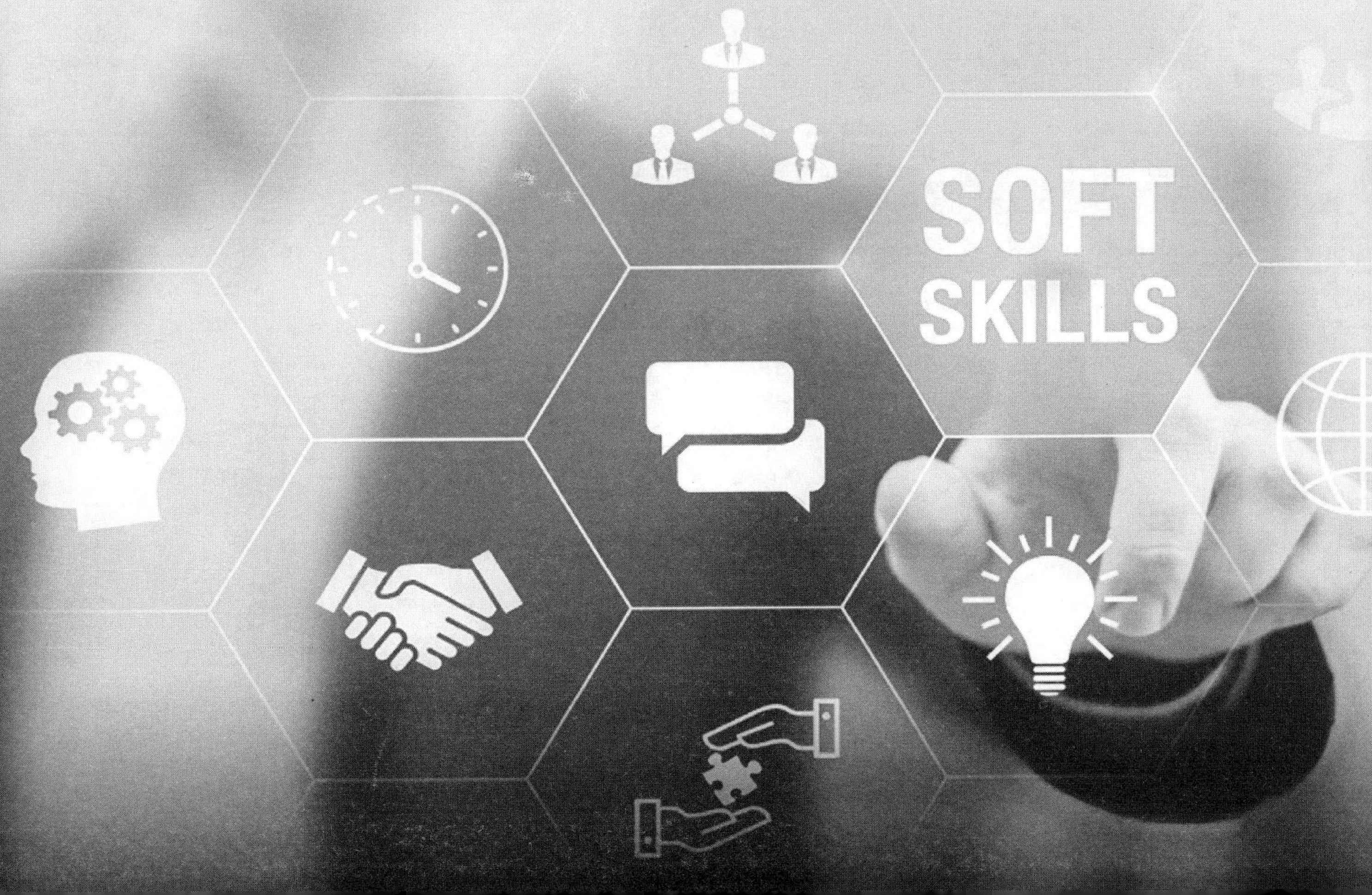

Attitude, Ethics and Communication (AETCOM)

PHASE II—MBBS

MODULE 2.1: THE FOUNDATIONS OF COMMUNICATION—2

Background

Communication is a fundamental prerequisite of the medical profession and beside skills is crucial in ensuring professional success for doctors. This module continues to provide an emphasis on effective communication skills. During professional year II, the emphasis is on active listening and data gathering.

Competencies Addressed

The student should be able to:	Level
1. Demonstrate ability to communicate to patients in a patient, respectful, non-threatening, non-judgmental and empathetic manner	SH

Learning Experience

- **Year of study:** Professional year 2
- **Hours:** 5 (1 + 2 + 1 + 1)
    1. Introductory small group session—1 hour
    2. Focused small group session—2 hours
    3. Skills lab session—1 hour
    4. Discussion and closure of case—1 hour.

Contents

- Introductory small group session on the principles of communication with focus on opening the discussion, listening and gathering data.
- Focused small group session with role play or videos where the students have an opportunity to observe, criticize and discuss common mistakes in opening the discussion, listening and data gathering.
- Skills lab sessions where students can perform tasks on standardized or regular patients with opportunity for self critique, critique by patient and by the facilitator.

Assessment

- **Formative:** Participation in session 2 and performance in session 3 may be used as part of formative assessment.
- **Summative:** May be deferred.

Resources

1. Makoul G. Essential elements of communication in medical encounters: The Kalamazoo consensus statement. Acad Med. 2001;76(4):390–3.
2. Hausberg M. Enhancing medical students' communication skills: Development and evaluation of an undergraduate training program. BMC Medical Education. 2012;12:16.

Note: Distribution of topics amongst the departments should be finalized by the concerned departments only.

REFLECTION: THE FOUNDATIONS OF COMMUNICATION—2

What happened:

....

....

....

....

....

....

So what:

....

....

....

....

....

....

What next:

....

....

....

....

....

Date   **Signature of Teacher-in-Charge**

MODULE 2.2: THE FOUNDATIONS OF BIOETHICS

Background

An introductory session in a large group that provides an overview of the evolution and the fundamental principles of bioethics including the cardinal pillars of ethics viz., autonomy, beneficence, non-malfeasance and justice.

Competencies Addressed

The student should be able to:	Level
1. Describe and discuss the role of non-malfeasance as a guiding principle in patient care	KH
2. Describe and discuss the role of autonomy and shared responsibility as a guiding principle in patient care	KH
3. Describe and discuss the role of beneficence of a guiding principle in patient care	KH
4. Describe and discuss the role of a physician in health care system	KH
5. Describe and discuss the role of justice as a guiding principle in patient care	KH

Learning Experience

- **Year of study:** Professional year 2
- **Hours:** 2 large group session—2 hours.

Contents

This module is a large group learning session that can be made interactive by illustrative examples.

Assessment

Summative: Short notes on—(a) Autonomy; (b) Beneficence; (c) Non-malfeasance.

Resource

1. A review of the four principles of bioethics is found here: http://archive.journalchirohumanities.com/Vol%20 14/JChioprHumanit 2007 v14_34-40.pdf.

REFLECTION ON: THE FOUNDATIONS OF BIOETHICS

What happened:

....

....

....

....

....

....

So what:

....

....

....

....

....

....

What next:

....

....

....

....

....

Date   **Signature of Teacher-in-Charge**

MODULE 2.3: HEALTH CARE AS A RIGHT

Background

This session is aimed at introducing students to health care systems, their access, equity in access, the impact of socioeconomic situations in determining health care access and the role of doctors as key players in the healthcare system.

Competencies Addressed

The student should be able to:	Level
1. Describe and discuss the role of justice as a guiding principle in patient care	KH

Learning Experience

- **Year of study:** Professional year 2
- **Hours:** 2
  1. Participatory student seminar—2 hours.

Contents

This module may be done as a participatory student seminar with debates on the more controversial issues to increase a reflective process.

Focus may be on:

1. Is health care a right?
2. What are the implications of health care as a right?
3. What are the social and economic implications of health care as a right?
4. What are the missing links? (see resource 2 for a brief overview) and
5. What are the implications for doctors?

Assessment

Summative: Short note on barriers to implementation of health care as a universal right.

Resources

1. The Universal Declaration of Human Rights. http://www.un.org/en/documents/udhr/
2. Missing links in universal health care. http://www.thehindu.com/opinion/lead/missing-links-in-universal-health-care/article6618667.ece

REFLECTION: HEALTH CARE AS A RIGHT

What happened:

....

....

....

....

....

....

....

So what:

....

....

....

....

....

....

What next:

....

....

....

....

....

Date   **Signature of Teacher-in-Charge**

MODULE 2.4: WORKING IN A HEALTH CARE TEAM

Background

This session is aimed at introducing students to health care systems and their functioning. It allows students to "tag along" with members of health care teams, observe their work and gain experience about their perspectives. It is hoped that this experience will help students to understand the need for collaborative work in health care, how each member of the health care team is important and also develop respect.

Competencies Addressed

The student should be able to:	Level
1. Demonstrate ability to work in a team of peers and superiors	SH
2. Demonstrate respect in relationship with patients, fellow team members, superiors and other health care workers	SH

Learning Experience

- **Year of study:** Professional year 2
- **Hours:** 6 hours (4 hours "tag along" + 2 hours discussion)
  1. "Tag along" session in hospital—2 × 2 hours
  2. Small group discussion session—2 hours.

Contents

This module may be done as two interdependent sessions:

1. A "tag along" session where students spend time with other health care workers including nurses, technicians and others, observe their work, their interactions, conduct a small interview with them and write a narrative based on this interview.
2. A small group discussion which is based on the students' observations, experiences, reflections and inferences and what must be done by them to work as an integral part of the health care team.

Assessment

Formative: Student participation in session 2 with assessment of submitted narrative.

REFLECTION: WORKING IN A HEALTHCARE TEAM

What happened:

....

....

....

....

....

....

So what:

....

....

....

....

....

....

What next:

....

....

....

....

....

....

Date   **Signature of Teacher-in-Charge**

MODULE 2.5: BIOETHICS CONTINUED—CASE STUDIES ON PATIENT AUTONOMY AND DECISION MAKING

Background

The important parts of ethical care of the patient are best learnt in a hybrid problem-based format with additional lectures and other sessions that allow students to learn collaboratively with different learning styles. A guide for case discussion is provided in the resources section of this module and may be used as a guide for other modules. The key element is that students remain in the same group with the same facilitator since groups mature in their learning over time.

Competencies Addressed

The student should be able to:	Level
1. Identify, discuss and defend medico-legal, socio-cultural and ethical issues as it pertains to patient autonomy, patient rights and shared responsibility in health care	KH

Learning Experience

- **Year of study:** Professional year 2
- **Hours:** 6
  1. Introduction and group formation—1 hour
  2. Case introduction—1 hour
  3. Self-directed learning—2 hours
  4. Anchoring lecture—1 hour
  5. Case resolution—1 hour

Case: The Cover Up

You evaluate Mrs Lakshmi Srinivasan who is a 48-year-old woman presenting with lymphadenopathy. She had been complaining of mild fever and weight loss for the past 4–5 months. Examination of the neck shows large rubbery lymph nodes that are present also in the axilla and the groin. There is a palpable spleen. She is accompanied by her caring husband.

Lakshmi undergoes a lymph node biopsy and the pathologist calls you and tells you that she has a lymphoma. That evening Mr. Srinivasan comes in first into your office and leaves the report on your table. As you read the description you realise that the final diagnosis has been altered to tuberculosis by whitening out the pathologist's report. When you look up he tells you—"Sir, I googled lymphoma—it is almost like a cancer. My wife can't handle that diagnosis. She has always been a worried frightened person. I want you to tell my wife that she had TB. She is waiting outside, doctor. I thought I will call her in after I had a chat about this with you".

Points for Discussion

1. Does the patient have a right to know their diagnosis?
2. What should the patient be told about their diagnosis, therapy and prognosis?
3. How much should be told to a patient about their illness?
4. Are there exceptions to full disclosure? Can family members request withholding of information from patient?

Assessment

- **Formative:** The student may be assessed based on their active participation in the sessions.
- **Summative:** Short questions on—
  1. Define patient autonomy.
  2. Contrast autonomy and paternalism.
  3. What are the responsibilities of patients and doctors in shared decision making?
  4. What is full and reasonable disclosure?

The suggested location, duration and requirements are as in item 2.

Once the case (or part of the case) is resolved, the next case (or the next part of the case) is introduced.

REFLECTION: BIOETHICS CONTINUED—CASE STUDIES ON PATIENT AUTONOMY AND DECISION MAKING

What happened:

....
....
....
....
....
....

So what:

....
....
....
....
....
....

What next:

....
....
....
....
....
....

Date   **Signature of Teacher-in-Charge**

MODULE 2.6: BIOETHICS CONTINUED—CASE STUDIES ON AUTONOMY AND DECISION MAKING
(Forensic Medicine and Toxicology)

Background

This introduces the student to further issues in autonomy including competence and capacity to make decisions (also see Module 2.5).

Competencies Addressed

The student should be able to:	Level
1. Identify, discuss and defend medico-legal, socio-cultural and ethical issues as they pertain to refusal of care including do not resuscitate and withdrawal of life support	KH

Learning Experience

- **Year of study:** Professional year 2
- **Hours:** 5
  1. Introduction of case—1 hour
  2. Self-directed learning —2 hours
  3. Anchoring lecture—1 hour
  4. Discussion and closure of case—1 hour.

Case: Life on a Machine

You are taking care of 78-year-old Mrs Mythili who was living all alone in an apartment with only a live-in caretaker, 3 streets away from your clinic. She is a widow and her only son emigrated to the US 32 years ago. He visits her once a year. One year ago, she had a fall with a hip fracture that healed badly. She has hypertension which is reasonably controlled on medications. She continues to come to your clinic once a month. Four months ago, she spent some time talking about her sister who recently died following metastatic breast cancer. "My sister suffered a lot, Doctor—they put a tube down her throat to breathe. Even when her heart stopped they kept thumping her chest—it was awful. If I ever fall sick I don't want to go through all this. Promise me, doctor, that you won't do all of this to me. I have lived all alone since my husband died but I have lived independently—now I don't want to depend on a machine to live". You had reassured her that she would be ok and this was just the recent death of her sister affecting her. On subsequent visits she would still bring up this issue and state that there was no use of her living as a burden to anyone and that no one should endure what her sister had undergone.

One day you get a call from the Emergency Room of the local hospital stating that Mrs Mythili has been admitted by the caretaker. She had developed fever and shortness of breath. She was brought hypoxic to the emergency room and they had intubated her. Chest X-ray revealed a large pneumonic patch. Laboratory testing revealed hyponatremia.

When you visited her she is somewhat drowsy, intubated and restrained. The nurse tells you that she is sometimes lucid; at other times not even able to recognise her son who was there since this morning. She points out at the ET and makes a pleading gesture to remove it. Her son accosts you in the hallway. He tells you that he got a call while he was traveling in Singapore and took the first flight out to be with his mom. He was very distressed at his mother's health and that he wants "everything" possible done for her. You ask him if she had ever indicated what she wanted to be done if she were to require hospitalization and intubation—he says that he used to speak to her every month on the phone and she was always cheerful and enquiring about her grandchildren but did not talk about her health.

Points for Discussion

1. Extent of patient autonomy.
2. Elements in decision making: Competency vs capacity.
3. Surrogacy in decision making.
4. Autonomy vs beneficence.
5. How much does family wishes count?
6. Legal, ethical and social aspects of 'Do not resuscitate'.

Assessment

- **Formative:** The student may be assessed based on their active participation in the sessions.
- **Summative:** Short questions on—(1) What determines decision making capacity and competency. (2) Who has the right to make decisions for a patient who cannot determine for himself.

Resources

See Module 2.5.

REFLECTION: BIOETHICS CONTINUED—CASE STUDIES ON AUTONOMY AND DECISION MAKING

What happened:

....
....
....
....
....
....

So what:

....
....
....
....
....
....
....

What next:

....
....
....
....
....

Date

Signature of Teacher-in-Charge

MODULE 2.7: BIOETHICS CONTINUED—CASE STUDIES ON AUTONOMY AND DECISION MAKING

Background

This introduces the student to further issues in autonomy including informed consent and refusal (also see Module 2.5).

Competencies Addressed

The student should be able to:	Level
1. Identify, discuss and defend, medico-legal, socio-cultural and ethical issues as they pertain to consent for surgical procedures	KH

Learning Experience

- **Year of study:** Professional year 2
- **Hours:** 5
    1. Introduction of case—1 hour
    2. Self-directed learning—2 hours
    3. Anchoring lecture—1 hour
    4. Discussion and closure of case—1 hour.

Case: Who is the Doctor?

A 54-year-old man named Mr Surendra Patel is admitted for acute chest pain in a medical centre. His father had died of a myocardial infarction at the age of 60. Two years ago, his brother had been admitted to a hospital with a myocardial infarction and had died after complications following an angioplasty. Mr Patel is a diabetic and is on multiple oral hypoglycemic agents with moderate control. He is a businessman with his own small industry. After initial stabilization, the patient is comfortable and pain-free after analgesics, nitrates and statins. Preliminary blood tests and ECG confirm an acute coronary event. The next morning, the senior cardiologist makes rounds and reviews the patient. "You have unstable angina, Mr Patel and require an angiogram. You may also require either a stent or coronary bypass after the procedure. The nurse will provide you with the necessary paperwork. Please sign it and I will plan the procedure for 4.35 AM tomorrow morning." "Doctor sahib", asked Mr Patel, "I am not comfortable with the idea of an angiogram; my brother died on the table when an angioplasty was being done. Aren't there other tests that you can do? I am not happy with this option". "Your brother would have had it with someone else, Mr Patel - I have the best hands in town; nothing will happen when I do it" retorted the cardiologist. "But aren't there any other options to see what I have? Is this the only test? I have read somewhere that you can do a CT angiogram", persisted Mr Patel. "Are you the doctor or am I the doctor?" retorted the cardiologist angrily. "If you are ready to do as I say, sign the papers and I will see you in the Cath lab tomorrow. Otherwise you are free to get discharged". He stomped out.

Points for Discussion

1. Extent of patient autonomy.
2. Informed consent and informed refusal.
3. Conflict between autonomy and beneficence.
4. What should the patient be told about a procedure?
5. What must the informed consent include?

Assessment

- **Formative:** The student may be assessed based on their active participation in the sessions.
- **Summative:** Short questions on—
    1. What is informed consent?
    2. What is informed refusal?

Resources

See Module 2.5.

REFLECTION: BIOETHICS CONTINUED—CASE STUDIES ON AUTONOMY AND DECISION MAKING

What happened:

....

....

....

....

....

....

So what:

....

....

....

....

....

....

....

What next:

....

....

....

....

....

....

Date   **Signature of Teacher-in-Charge**

MODULE 2.8: WHAT DOES IT MEAN TO BE FAMILY MEMBER OF A SICK PATIENT?

Background

Doctors deal with human suffering throughout their professional careers. A balanced approach to the patient care experience requires an understanding of support systems of patients, priorities coping and emotions of families, the role of the doctor, an exploration of empathy vs equanimity and the difference between healing and curing and support.

Competencies Addressed

The student should be able to:	Level
1. Demonstrate empathy in patient encounters	SH

Learning Experience

- **Year of study:** Professional year 2
- **Hours:** 6 (includes 2 hours of SDL)
  1. Hospital visit and interviews—2 hours
     - Students are assigned to patients in the *hospital, interview their family about their illnesses, experience, reactions, emotions, outlook and expectations* or can be done in a controlled environment with standardised patients.
  2. Large group discussions with patients' relatives—1 hour
     - Family members of patients with different illnesses may be brought to a large group discussion with permission and an interactive discussion (based on the items outlined in Session 1. Can use standardized patients)
  3. Self-directed learning—2 hours
     - Self-directed learning where students write a report from reflection based on Sessions 1 and 2 and on other readings, TV series, movies, etc.
  4. Discussion and closure—1 hour.
     - A closure session with students to share their reflections based on 1, 2 and 3 so that it includes how they intend to incorporate the lessons learnt in patient care.

Assessment

- **Formative:** The student may be assessed based on their active participation in the sessions and submission of the written narrative.
- **Summative:** Short questions on the role of doctors in the community and expectations of society form doctors, e.g.—
  1. What is empathy? What is the role of empathy in the care of patients?

REFLECTION: WHAT DOES IT MEAN TO BE FAMILY MEMBER OF A SICK PATIENT?

What happened:

....

....

....

....

....

....

So what:

....

....

....

....

....

....

What next:

....

....

....

....

....

....

Date   **Signature of Teacher-in-Charge**

PHASE III—PART I MBBS

MODULE 3.1: THE FOUNDATIONS OF COMMUNICATION—3

Background

Communication is a fundamental prerequisite of the medical profession and beside skills is crucial in ensuring professional success for doctors. This module builds on the listening skills developed in professional year II. The Kalamazoo consensus statement provides a working model of teaching communication skills and may be used to impart communication skills. Skills, that will be introduced, should include "dealing with emotion".

Competency Addressed

The student should be able to:	Level
1. Demonstrate ability to communicate to patients in a patient, respectful, non-threatening, non-judgmental and empathetic manner	SH

Learning Experience

- **Year of study:** Professional year 3
- **Hours:** 5 (1 + 2 + 2)
    1. Introductory small group session—1 hour
    2. Focused small group session—2 hours
    3. Skills lab session—2 hours.

Contents

- Introductory small group session on the principles of communication with focus on dealing with emotions.
- Focused small group session with role play or video where students have an opportunity to observe, critique and discuss common mistakes when dealing with emotion.
- Skills lab sessions where students can perform tasks on standardised or regular patients with opportunity for self critique, critique by patient and by facilitator.

Assessment

- **Formative:** Participation in session 2 and performance in session 3 may be used as part of formative assessment.
- **Summative:** May be deferred.

Resources

1. Makoul G. Essential elements of communication in medical encounters: The Kalamazoo consensus statement. Acad Med. 2001;76(4):390–3.
2. Hausberg M. Enhancing medical students' communication skills: Development and evaluation of an undergraduate training program. BMC Medical Education. 2012;12:16.

REFLECTION: THE FOUNDATIONS OF COMMUNICATION—3

What happened:

....

....

....

....

....

....

So what:

....

....

....

....

....

....

What next:

....

....

....

....

....

....

Date   **Signature of Teacher-in-Charge**

MODULE 3.2: CASE STUDIES IN BIOETHICS—DISCLOSURE OF MEDICAL ERRORS

Background

This introduces the student to further issues in autonomy including full disclosure of mistakes (also see Module 2.5).

Competency Addressed

The student should be able to:	Level
1. Demonstrate an understanding of the implications and the appropriate procedure and response to be followed in the event of medical errors	SH

Learning Experience

- **Year of study:** Professional year 3
- **Hours:** 5
  1. Introduction of case—1 hour
  2. Self-directed learning—2 hours
  3. Anchoring lecture—1 hour
  4. Discussion and closure of case—1 hour.

Case: Seeking Immunity

It was a busy clinic day and getting worse. Patients were getting impatient. Time was marching and details were becoming a casualty. Five year old Madhumita comes in with her mother. She has asthma and is under your care. You examine her and adjust your prescriptions and start your good byes. At that time, her mother reminds you that she is due for her booster shots. Oh that, you frown—and tell her to wait for a few minutes and that you will have the nurse load the injection and come to the adjoining room and give the injection. You ask the nurse to load the injection and keep it for you over the intercom.

You continue to see patients. After a couple of patients, the mother knocks indicating that she is getting late. You get up and go to the next room. The nurse is not there but you find a loaded syringe. You quickly administer the injection to the child and get back to seeing patients.

A few minutes later, the nurse calls back saying that she has loaded Madhumita's injections. You drop everything and go into the injection room and confront the nurse "But doctor that was gentamicin I had loaded for Mrs Asif" she says.

Points for Discussion

1. Medical errors in clinical care.
2. The correct approach to disclosure of medical errors.
3. Consequence of failure to disclosure of medical errors including medico-legal, social and loss of trust.

Assessment

- **Formative:** The student may be assessed based on their active participation in the sessions including role play on disclosure of errors.
- **Summative:** Short questions on—What is the ethical standard in dealing with medical errors?

REFLECTION: CASE STUDIES IN BIOETHICS—DISCLOSURE OF MEDICAL ERRORS

What happened:

....

....

....

....

....

....

So what:

....

....

....

....

....

....

What next:

....

....

....

....

....

Date   **Signature of Teacher-in-Charge**

MODULE 3.3: THE FOUNDATIONS OF COMMUNICATION—4

Background

Communication is a fundamental prerequisite of the medical profession and beside skills is crucial in ensuring professional success for doctors. This module continues to provide an emphasis on effective communication skills. The emphasis is on administering informed consent during professional year III.

Competencies Addressed

The student should be able to:	Level
1. Demonstrate ability to communicate to patients in a patient, respectful, nonthreatening, non-judgmental and empathetic manner	SH
2. Identify, discuss and defend, medico-legal, socio-cultural and ethical issues as they pertain to consent for surgical procedures	KH
3. Administer informed consent and appropriately address patient queries to a patient undergoing a surgical procedure in a simulated environment	SH

Learning Experience

- **Year of study:** Professional year 3
- **Hours:** 5 (1 + 2 + 2)
  1. Introductory small group session—1 hour
  2. Focused small group session—2 hours
  3. Skills Lab session—2 hours.

Contents

- Introductory small group session on the principles of communication with focus on administering informed consent.
- Focused small group session with role play or video where students have an opportunity to observe, criticise and discuss common mistakes in administering informed consent.
- Skills lab sessions where students can perform tasks on standardised or regular patients with opportunity for self critique, critique by patient and by facilitator.

Assessment

- **Formative:** Participation in session 2 and performance in session 3 may be used as part of formative assessment.
- **Summative:** A skill station in which the student may administer informed consent to a standardized patient.

Resources

1. Makoul G. Essential elements of communication in medical encounters: The Kalamazoo consensus statement. Acad Med. 2001;76(4):390-3.
2. Hausberg M. Enhancing medical students' communication skills: Development and evaluation of an undergraduate training program. BMC Medical Education. 2012;12:16.

REFLECTION: THE FOUNDATIONS OF COMMUNICATION—4

What happened:

So what:

What next:

Date   **Signature of Teacher-in-Charge**

MODULE 3.4: CASE STUDIES IN BIOETHICS—CONFIDENTIALITY
(Forensic Medicine and Toxicology)

Background

This introduces the student to confidentiality and its limits (also see Module 2.5).

Competency Addressed

The student should be able to:	Level
1. Identify, discuss and defend medico-legal, socio-cultural and ethical issues as it pertains to confidentiality in patient care	KH

Learning Experience

- **Year of study:** Professional year 3
- **Hours:** 5
  1. Introduction of case—1 hour
  2. Self-directed learning—2 hours
  3. Anchoring lecture—1 hour
  4. Discussion and closure of case—1 hour.

Case: Do Not Tell My Wife

Ramratan was in tears. "How is it possible doctor? We are expecting our son soon. He will not have a father". Ramratan had seen you with vague aches, fever, weight loss and cough with expectoration not responsive to antibiotics for the past three months. He had a right mid zone lung shadow on X-ray and the sputum was positive for AFB. On being questioned, he had revealed that he had unprotected sexual intercourse with multiple partners 3 years ago. "But I stopped after I married Danno, doctor—I am faithful to her". An informed consent was obtained and HIV screening test was ordered and it was positive. A confirmatory test was subsequently obtained and it was also positive. The CDC count was < 100. Ramratan had come to discuss the results of his HIV test. After consoling him and writing out prescriptions for TB and HIV, you mention to him that he must bring his wife for testing. "This is important, Ramratan", you add - "especially since she is pregnant."

"Absolutely not, sir!" he explosively retorts. "That is not possible. I will be humiliated. Danno will leave me and go. I will never be able to see my son. I will become an outcast in our community. I can't live without my wife, doctor. I urge you, doctor—don't do this. I forbid you".

Points for Discussion

1. The primacy of confidentiality in patient care.
2. What does confidentiality entail?
3. When can confidence be breached with whom and how?
4. Confidentiality and diseases that may engender patients and society.

Assessment

- **Formative:** The student may be assessed based on their active participation in the sessions.
- **Summative:** Short questions on—
  - What are the instances in which confidentiality of patient information may be breached?

REFLECTION: CASE STUDIES IN BIOETHICS—CONFIDENTIALITY

What happened:

So what:

What next:

Date   **Signature of Teacher-in-Charge**

MODULE 3.5: CASE STUDIES IN BIOETHICS—FIDUCIARY DUTY

Background

This module discusses doctor's duty including fiduciary duty (also see Module 2.5).

Competencies Addressed

The student should be able to:	Level
1. Identify, discuss and defend medico-legal, socio-cultural, professional and ethical issues as it pertains to the physician - patient relationship (including fiduciary duty)	KH
2. Identify and discuss physician's role and responsibility to society and the community that she/he serves	KH

Learning Experience

- **Year of study:** Professional year 3
- **Hours:** 5
    1. Introduction of case—1 hour
    2. Self-directed learning—2 hours
    3. Anchoring lecture—1 hour
    4. Discussion and closure of case—1 hour.

Case: Is He a Human Being or a Machine?

It was a long day and the surgeon has finished four surgeries. Two of these were complicated surgeries requiring all his experience and skills. But it was gratifying. After that he had seen 40 outpatients. He was the most successful doctor in that small community and had provided service for the past 25 years. He had finished his outpatient, ate his meal and went to bed. The night duty doctor who usually comes around 10 pm to sit in the clinic and answer calls from inpatients had taken the night off - he had entrance exams next day. Praying it would be a quiet night he told his wife - I am very very tired; make sure that I am not disturbed.

He woke up at 1 AM with the sounds of commotion downstairs. He could hear signs of arguing - Call the doctor, he must come down. He could hear his wife—"please take her to the nearest government hospital. This is a surgical nursing home and doctor is very tired—I cannot wake him up." He could hear irate patient attendants—"but your board says open 24 hours for emergency. The town hospital is 15 km. away. I don't know if my daughter will make it. By the time the venom will reach the brain. Call your husband now madam. This is not correct". His wife retorted "He has worked from 4 AM this morning—he has gone to sleep very tired asking me not to wake him up. Is he the only doctor in town? Is he a human being or a machine? Why are you being unreasonable?" The surgeon reached out for his clothe.

Points for Discussion

1. Duty of a doctor.
2. The concept of fiduciary duty.
3. Balancing personal and professional life.
4. Where to draw the line!

Assessment

- **Formative:** The student may be assessed based on their active participation in the sessions.
- **Summative:** Short questions on—
    - What is fiduciary duty?

REFLECTION: CASE STUDIES IN BIOETHICS—FIDUCIARY DUTY

What happened:

....

....

....

....

....

....

So what:

....

....

....

....

....

....

What next:

....

....

....

....

....

....

Date   **Signature of Teacher-in-Charge**

4

Simulation Based Teaching (Skill Lab), Vertical Integration and Seminar

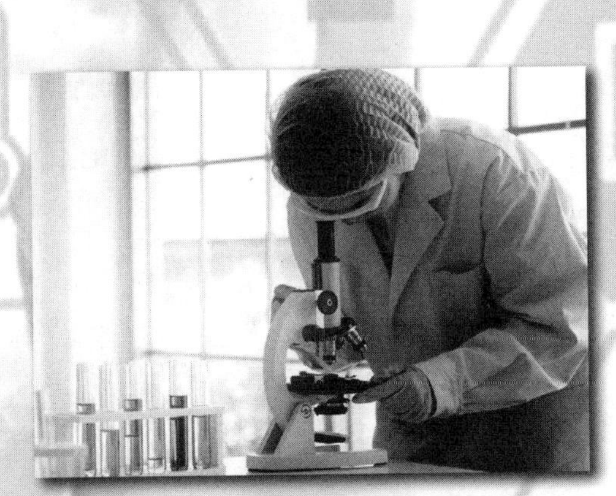

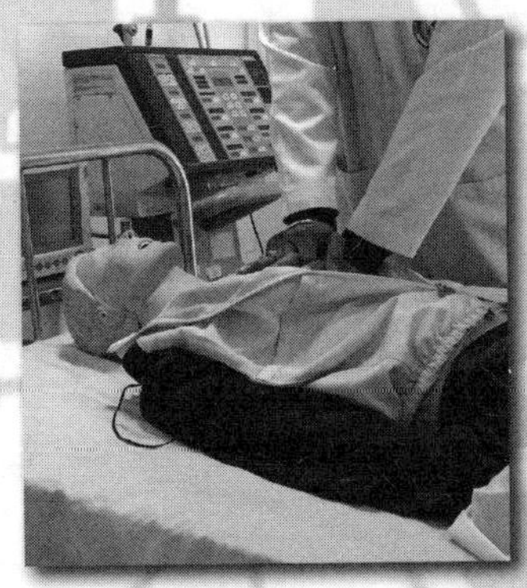

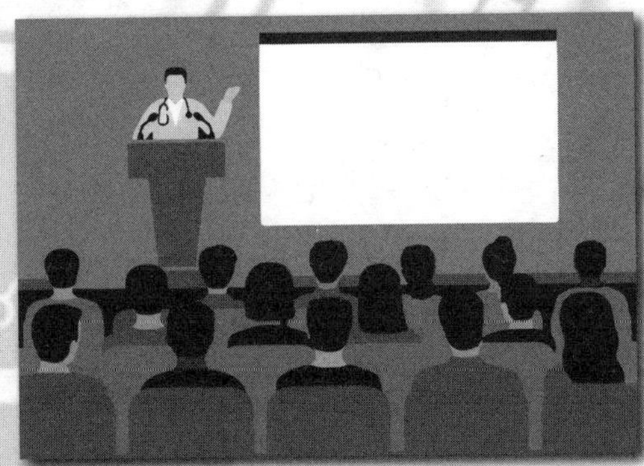

Skill Lab, Vertical Integration and Seminar

RECORD SHEET OF SKILL LAB/VERTICAL INTEGRATION/SEMINAR

Sl. No.	Topic	Competency addressed	Name of the activity	Date completed (dd-mm-yyyy)	Attempt at activity	Rating	Decision of faculty	Faculty initials	Feedback received
					First only (F) Repeat (R) Remedial (Re)	Below (B) expectations Meets (M) expectations Exceeds (E) expectations or numerical scores	Completed (C) Repeat (R) Remedial (Re)		Initial of learner

REFLECTION: SKILL LAB

Topic: **Date:**

What happened:

So what:

What next:

Signature of Teacher-in-charge

REFLECTION: SKILL LAB

Topic: **Date:**

What happened:

So what:

What next:

Signature of Teacher-in-charge

REFLECTION: SKILL LAB

Topic: **Date:**

What happened:

So what:

What next:

                                                                        Signature of Teacher-in-charge

REFLECTION: SKILL LAB

Topic: **Date:**

What happened:

So what:

What next:

                                                                        Signature of Teacher-in-charge

REFLECTION: VERTICAL INTEGRATION

Topic: **Date:**

What happened:

So what:

What next:

Signature of Teacher-in-charge

REFLECTION: VERTICAL INTEGRATION

Topic: **Date:**

What happened:

So what:

What next:

Signature of Teacher-in-charge

REFLECTION: VERTICAL INTEGRATION

Topic: **Date:**

What happened:

So what:

What next:

                                                                 Signature of Teacher-in-charge

REFLECTION: VERTICAL INTEGRATION

Topic: **Date:**

What happened:

So what:

What next:

                                                                 Signature of Teacher-in-charge

REFLECTION: SEMINAR

Topic: **Date:**

What happened:

So what:

What next:

                                                                        Signature of Teacher-in-charge

REFLECTION: SEMINAR

Topic: **Date:**

What happened:

So what:

What next:

                                                                        Signature of Teacher-in-charge

REFLECTION: SEMINAR

Topic: **Date:**

What happened:

So what:

What next:

Signature of Teacher-in-charge

REFLECTION: SEMINAR

Topic: **Date:**

What happened:

So what:

What next:

Signature of Teacher-in-charge